ANTI-INFLAMMATORY DIET
FOR BEGINNERS

Asher Greenfield

Disclaimer Notice

The author of this book and its publishers have made every effort to ensure that the information provided is accurate and up-to-date at the time of publication. However, medical knowledge is constantly evolving, and new research can alter the understanding of health and nutrition. Therefore, the author and the publisher cannot guarantee the accuracy, completeness, or timeliness of the information presented within this book.

The Anti-Inflammatory Diet outlined in this book is a dietary approach that may have potential health benefits, but its suitability for individuals may vary. It is essential to consult with a healthcare professional before making any significant changes to your diet, especially if you have any underlying health conditions, allergies, or are taking medications.

The author and the publisher disclaim any responsibility for any adverse effects or consequences resulting from the use or application of the information contained in this book. The reader assumes full responsibility for their actions and decisions regarding their health and diet, and the author and publisher are not liable for any direct or indirect damages or losses that may arise.

Table of Contents

Introduction..5
Chapter 1: Understanding Inflammation.. 6
   The Basics of Inflammation..6
   Chronic vs. Acute Inflammation...7
   Signs and Symptoms of Chronic Inflammation...8
   Inflammatory Foods to Avoid...9
   Anti-Inflammatory Foods to Embrace..11
Chapter 2: Planning Your Anti-Inflammatory Journey...................................... 13
   Setting Your Goals..13
   Creating a Grocery List...15
   Stocking Your Kitchen...17
   Meal Prep Tips..18
Chapter 3: The 28-Day Meal Plan... 20
   Day-by-Day Detox Meal Plan..20
   Staying on Track: Week 5 and Beyond...30
Chapter 4: Delicious Anti-Inflammatory Recipes..31
   Breakfast Recipes...31
      Turmeric Scrambled Eggs..31
      Chia Seed Pudding...32
      Avocado Toast..33
      Oatmeal with Berries..34
      Greek Yogurt Parfait...35
      Quinoa Breakfast Bowl..36
      Smoothie Bowl...37
      Ginger-Tahini Buckwheat Pancakes...38
      Sweet Potato Hash...39
      Spinach and Mushroom Omelette...40
      Berry Breakfast Quinoa...41
      Savory Quinoa Porridge..42
      Shakshuka with Spinach and Bell Peppers...43
      Buckwheat Porridge with Almond Butter and Fresh Figs.......................44
   Lunch Recipes..45
      Salmon Salad...45
      Quinoa and Black Bean Bowl..46
      Grilled Chicken and Quinoa Bowl..47
      Mediterranean Tuna Wrap...48
      Crispy Bass with Citrus Soba..49
      Chicken and Kale Caesar Salad..50
      Cauliflower Rice Bowl..51
      Caprese Quinoa Salad..52
      Spicy Black Bean and Sweet Potato Bowl...53
      Zucchini Noodles with Pesto...54
      Turkey and Avocado Lettuce Wraps..55
      Veggie Stir-Fry...56
      Baked Cod with Roasted Root Vegetables...57
      Mediterranean Grilled Fish with Spaghetti...58

Dinner Recipes...59
    Baked Salmon with Asparagus...59
    Shrimp Cauliflower Rice Skillet..60
    Turmeric Chickpea Curry...61
    Grilled Vegetable and Quinoa Stuffed Peppers................................62
    Creamy Lemon-Spinach Spaghetti..63
    Lemon Herb Baked Chicken...64
    Spiced Lentil and Vegetable Soup..65
    Baked Spinach and Feta Pasta...66
    Tofu and Vegetable Stir-Fry...67
    Baked Eggplant with Tomato and Almond Topping...........................68
    Spaghetti Squash with Pesto...69
    Grilled Shrimp and Pineapple Skewers..70
    Chopped Power Salad with Chicken..71
    Eggs with Tomato, Chickpeas and Spinach....................................72
Snack Recipes..73
    Cucumber and Hummus..73
    Greek Yogurt and Berries..74
    Trail Mix...75
    Carrot Sticks with Guacamole..76
    Kale Chips..77
    Almonds and Dark Chocolate...78
    Apple Slices with Almond Butter...79
    Peanut Butter Energy Balls..80
    Roasted Chickpeas..81
    Sliced Bell Peppers with Salsa...82
Chapter 5: Beyond the Diet...**83**
The Role of Exercise..83
Managing Stress..85
Quality Sleep..87
Staying Hydrated...89
Tracking Your Progress...90
Chapter 6: Common Questions and Concerns......................................**91**
Dining Out While on an Anti-Inflammatory Diet...91
Dealing with Food Allergies..93
Budget-Friendly Anti-Inflammatory Eating..95
Sustainability and Eco-Friendly Choices..97
Chapter 7: Resources and References...**99**
Websites and Apps...99
Further Assistance...101
Conclusion...**102**
Appendices..**103**
Glossary of Anti-Inflammatory Terms...103
Measurement Conversion Charts...104
Personal Notes...**106**

Introduction

The Anti-Inflammatory Diet isn't just a fad or a passing trend – it's a scientifically-backed way to address one of the root causes of various chronic diseases. Inflammation, while essential for healing acute injuries and infections, can become problematic when it becomes chronic. This persistent, low-level inflammation is associated with a host of health issues, including heart disease, diabetes, arthritis, and even some cancers. By adopting an Anti-Inflammatory Diet, individuals can harness the power of nutrition to help combat this hidden enemy within their bodies.

To fully appreciate the importance of the Anti-Inflammatory Diet, one must first comprehend the intricacies of chronic inflammation. Inflammation is the body's natural response to injury and stress, but when it persists for extended periods without a clear threat to combat, it can become destructive. The biochemical processes involved in chronic inflammation can damage cells, tissues, and organs, leading to a wide range of health problems. By reducing the triggers of chronic inflammation through dietary choices, individuals can regain control over their health.

The benefits of embracing an Anti-Inflammatory Diet are far-reaching. Beyond simply reducing inflammation, this dietary approach offers numerous advantages that can enhance one's quality of life. From weight management and improved energy levels to better mental clarity and a reduced risk of chronic diseases, the Anti-Inflammatory Diet is a holistic solution to achieving optimal health and vitality.

While the Anti-Inflammatory Diet holds the potential to benefit everyone, this book is designed with a specific audience in mind. It is for those who may have heard about the Anti-Inflammatory Diet but are unsure of where to start. It's for individuals who want to take control of their health, reduce the risk of chronic diseases, and enjoy a vibrant, energetic life. Whether you're a complete beginner to the concept or someone looking for practical guidance, this book is tailored to your needs.

This book is not just a collection of ideas and theories; it's a practical guide for real-life application. To help readers make the most of this resource, we've included step-by-step instructions, meal plans, recipes, and tools to facilitate your journey towards a healthier, less inflamed life. In the following sections, you'll find comprehensive information on the Anti-Inflammatory Diet, a 28-Day Detox Plan, and a wide array of delicious recipes that will make adopting this lifestyle a pleasurable and sustainable experience.

Chapter 1: Understanding Inflammation

The Basics of Inflammation

Inflammation is a natural and essential process that occurs within our bodies in response to various stimuli. It's a part of the body's defense mechanism, designed to protect us from harmful invaders like bacteria, viruses, and toxins. While acute inflammation is necessary for our survival, chronic inflammation can be detrimental to our health. Understanding the basics of inflammation is a key component of embracing an anti-inflammatory diet.

Inflammatory Foods and Lifestyle Factors

Several factors contribute to chronic inflammation, with diet and lifestyle playing a significant role. These include:

Diet: Some foods can promote inflammation, while others have anti-inflammatory properties. Highly processed foods, sugary beverages, and saturated fats can fuel inflammation, whereas fruits, vegetables, whole grains, and fatty fish like salmon can help reduce it. We'll delve deeper into these dietary choices later in the book.

Stress: Chronic stress can trigger an inflammatory response in your body. Learning stress management techniques, such as mindfulness, meditation, and exercise, is crucial for managing inflammation.

Lack of Physical Activity: A sedentary lifestyle is associated with chronic inflammation. Regular exercise, on the other hand, can have anti-inflammatory effects.

Sleep: Poor sleep quality or insufficient sleep can exacerbate inflammation. It's essential to prioritize good sleep habits.

Environmental Factors: Exposure to pollutants and toxins in the environment can contribute to inflammation. Minimizing exposure and making eco-friendly choices can help.

Balancing Inflammation

Understanding the balance between acute and chronic inflammation is key. Acute inflammation is necessary for healing, but chronic inflammation is something we want to minimize. Your anti-inflammatory diet and lifestyle changes will focus on reducing chronic inflammation while allowing your body to effectively respond to acute inflammation when necessary.

In the following chapters, we will explore in detail the foods, habits, and strategies that can help you manage inflammation and enjoy the many health benefits of an anti-inflammatory diet.

Chronic vs. Acute Inflammation

To fully comprehend the significance of an anti-inflammatory diet, it's crucial to distinguish between two primary types of inflammation: acute and chronic inflammation. These distinct forms of inflammation serve different purposes in the body and have contrasting effects on your health.

Acute Inflammation	Chronic Inflammation
Acute inflammation is a fundamental and immediate response by your immune system to a specific threat or injury. It's a protective mechanism that plays a vital role in the healing process. When you cut your finger, sprain an ankle, or catch a cold, acute inflammation kicks in to combat the problem. Here are some key characteristics of acute inflammation: **Short-Term Nature:** Acute inflammation typically occurs for a short duration, often a matter of days or a few weeks at most. **Clear Symptoms:** Acute inflammation is associated with visible signs, including redness, swelling, heat, and pain. These symptoms are indicative of the immune system at work. **Purposeful Response:** It's the body's way of isolating and eliminating harmful agents, promoting tissue repair, and defending against infections. **Resolution:** After the threat is neutralized, acute inflammation gradually subsides, allowing the body to return to its normal state. **Necessary for Healing:** Without acute inflammation, wounds wouldn't heal, and infections could become life-threatening.	Chronic inflammation, on the other hand, is an ongoing, low-level inflammation that persists for an extended period, often without noticeable symptoms. This type of inflammation can be damaging and is linked to a variety of health problems. Here's what sets chronic inflammation apart: **Long-Term Presence:** Chronic inflammation can linger for weeks, months, or even years, slowly wearing down your body. **Subtle or Absent Symptoms:** Unlike acute inflammation, chronic inflammation often goes unnoticed, making it a silent contributor to health issues. **Underlying Health Conditions:** Chronic inflammation is associated with various chronic diseases, including heart disease, diabetes, arthritis, and even cancer. **Lifestyle and Environmental Factors:** Diet, stress, lack of exercise, and environmental toxins are known to fuel chronic inflammation. **Destabilizing Effect:** Chronic inflammation can lead to damage to healthy tissues and contribute to the development and progression of chronic diseases.

In summary, while acute inflammation is a necessary part of your body's defense and healing mechanisms, chronic inflammation is problematic and requires attention to mitigate its adverse effects. An anti-inflammatory diet primarily aims to reduce chronic inflammation by minimizing the factors that contribute to its development.

Understanding the difference between these two types of inflammation is pivotal in adopting dietary and lifestyle changes that can help you better manage your health and well-being.

Signs and Symptoms of Chronic Inflammation

Persistent Fatigue	Feeling persistently tired and drained could be a sign of chronic inflammation. When the body is in a state of chronic inflammation, it releases cytokines and other immune molecules that can disrupt the body's natural energy production processes.
Unexplained Weight Gain	Chronic inflammation can lead to weight gain, especially around the midsection. This is due to the release of inflammatory molecules that interfere with insulin sensitivity and encourage the storage of fat.
Joint Pain	Inflammation of the joints is a hallmark of conditions like rheumatoid arthritis. However, chronic inflammation can also lead to joint pain and stiffness, even without an autoimmune disorder. This can sometimes be mistaken for the normal signs of aging.
Skin Problems	Skin issues like acne, eczema, and psoriasis are often related to chronic inflammation. Inflammation can disrupt the normal function of skin cells and cause various dermatological problems.
Gastrointestinal Distress	Chronic inflammation in the gut can lead to digestive problems such as bloating, gas, diarrhea, and even conditions like irritable bowel syndrome (IBS). It can also disrupt the balance of gut bacteria, leading to dysbiosis.
Cognitive Decline	Inflammation may contribute to cognitive decline and an increased risk of neurodegenerative diseases like Alzheimer's. People with chronic inflammation may experience brain fog, forgetfulness, and difficulties with concentration.
Allergies and Sensitivities	Chronic inflammation can exacerbate allergies and food sensitivities, making them more severe and difficult to manage. It can also contribute to the development of new allergies over time.
Autoimmune Diseases	In cases of autoimmune diseases like lupus, Crohn's disease, and multiple sclerosis, the body's immune system mistakenly attacks healthy tissues. Chronic inflammation plays a significant role in triggering and perpetuating these conditions.

Inflammatory Foods to Avoid

Understanding which foods promote inflammation is crucial for maintaining a balanced, anti-inflammatory diet. Below is a comprehensive guide to the main categories of inflammatory foods you should consider avoiding.

Processed Meats: Processed meats, including sausages, hot dogs, bacon, and deli meats, are high in saturated fats, nitrates, and preservatives. These substances can trigger inflammatory responses in the body, increasing the risk of cardiovascular diseases and certain cancers. Regular consumption of processed meats has also been linked to metabolic disturbances.

Refined Carbohydrates: Refined carbohydrates, such as white bread, white rice, pastries, and many breakfast cereals, have been stripped of their natural fiber and nutrients. This leads to rapid spikes in blood sugar levels, which can promote inflammation. High intake of refined carbs is associated with an increased risk of obesity, insulin resistance, and inflammatory diseases.

Sugary Foods and Drinks: Foods and beverages high in added sugars, like sodas, candies, desserts, and sweetened beverages, can lead to chronic inflammation. Excessive sugar intake stimulates the production of pro-inflammatory cytokines and contributes to insulin resistance, obesity, and other metabolic issues.

Fried Foods: Fried foods, including French fries, fried chicken, and doughnuts, often contain high levels of unhealthy fats and advanced glycation end products (AGEs), which can trigger inflammation. These foods also contribute to weight gain, which further exacerbates inflammatory responses in the body.

Trans Fats and Unhealthy Oils: Trans fats, commonly found in margarine, processed snacks, baked goods, and some fast foods, are known to promote inflammation. Additionally, oils high in omega-6 fatty acids, such as corn, soybean, and sunflower oils, can disrupt the balance of fatty acids in the body and lead to inflammatory processes when consumed in excess.

Artificial Ingredients: Artificial sweeteners, colorings, flavor enhancers (like monosodium glutamate or MSG), and preservatives can provoke inflammatory reactions in sensitive individuals. While not everyone reacts the same way, minimizing exposure to these additives is advisable for maintaining an anti-inflammatory lifestyle.

High-Sodium Foods: Excessive sodium intake from processed foods, canned soups, salty snacks, and fast food can contribute to inflammation and elevate blood pressure. High sodium levels can also impair the function of the endothelial cells lining the blood vessels, leading to vascular inflammation.

Alcoholic Beverages: While moderate alcohol consumption may have some health benefits, excessive intake can cause systemic inflammation. Alcohol can irritate the gastrointestinal tract, alter gut microbiota, and increase the permeability of the intestinal lining, allowing inflammatory toxins to enter the bloodstream.

Foods to Avoid

Processed and Packaged Foods:

- Fast food (burgers, fries, chicken nuggets)
- Packaged snacks (chips, crackers, salted snacks)
- Frozen meals (frozen pizza, lasagna, ready-to-eat dinners)
- Instant noodles and canned pasta
- Processed meats (sausages, bacon, ham, smoked meats)

Refined Carbohydrates:

- White bread and white rice
- Pasta made with refined flour
- Pastries and baked goods (croissants, donuts, muffins)
- Sweet breakfast cereals

Sugary Foods and Beverages:

- Soda and sweetened soft drinks
- Fruit juices with added sugar
- Candy and chocolate bars with high sugar content
- Desserts (cakes, pies, cookies, ice cream)

Unhealthy Fats:

- Trans fats (margarine, shortening, store-bought baked goods)
- Deep-fried foods (French fries, fried chicken, onion rings)
- Processed snacks with hydrogenated oils
- Fatty cuts of red meat (ribeye, pork belly)

Processed Oils High in Omega-6:

- Safflower oil
- Corn oil
- Soybean oil
- Cottonseed oil
- Sunflower oil

High-Sodium Foods:

- Processed meats (deli meats, bacon, sausages)
- Canned soups and vegetables with added salt
- Pickles and salty snacks (salted nuts, crackers)
- Ready-made sauces and dressings

Gluten-Containing Grains (for Gluten-Sensitive Individuals):

- Wheat (bread, pasta, pastries)
- Barley (malt products, beer)
- Rye (rye bread, cereals)
- Spelt and other ancient grains containing gluten

Dairy Products:

- Whole milk, cream, and butter
- Full-fat cheeses (cheddar, brie)
- Flavored yogurts with added sugars
- Sweetened condensed milk

High-Glycemic Index Foods:

- White bread and refined pasta
- Instant oatmeal
- Rice cakes and puffed cereals
- Pretzels and bagels

Alcohol:

- Beer
- Wine
- Spirits (vodka, whiskey, rum)
- Sugary cocktails

Artificial Additives and Preservatives:

- Artificial sweeteners (aspartame, saccharin, sucralose)
- Food colorings (Red 40, Yellow 5, Blue 1)
- Flavor enhancers (monosodium glutamate - MSG)
- Preservatives (sodium nitrite, BHA, BHT)

Anti-Inflammatory Foods to Embrace

Now that you're aware of the inflammatory foods to avoid, it's equally important to understand which foods can help reduce chronic inflammation and promote overall well-being. These anti-inflammatory foods should be a fundamental part of your diet:

Prioritize Fruits and Vegetables: Fruits and vegetables are the foundation of an anti-inflammatory diet. They are rich in vitamins, minerals, fiber, and antioxidants that help neutralize free radicals and combat oxidative stress. Aim to fill half of your plate with a variety of colorful fruits and vegetables at each meal. The diversity in color reflects a range of beneficial nutrients, so incorporating greens, reds, yellows, and purples ensures a broad spectrum of health benefits.

Focus on Healthy Fats: Incorporating healthy fats, especially omega-3 fatty acids, is crucial. These fats help regulate inflammation in the body and support heart and brain health. Replace saturated and trans fats with sources of unsaturated fats, such as extra virgin olive oil, avocados, and nuts. Regular consumption of fatty fish is also recommended to boost omega-3 intake.

Choose Whole Grains Over Refined Grains: Whole grains retain their natural fiber, vitamins, and minerals, which help stabilize blood sugar levels and reduce inflammation. Instead of refined grains like white bread and pasta, opt for whole grains such as oats, quinoa, and brown rice. Their high fiber content also supports gut health, which plays a role in managing inflammation.

Include Lean Proteins: Proteins are essential for maintaining muscle mass and supporting bodily functions. Choose lean protein sources, such as skinless poultry, legumes, and plant-based proteins like tofu and tempeh. These options provide necessary nutrients without the inflammatory effects often associated with red and processed meats.

Embrace Fermented and Probiotic-Rich Foods: A healthy gut microbiome is linked to lower inflammation levels. Incorporate fermented foods like yogurt, kefir, sauerkraut, and kimchi to promote beneficial gut bacteria. A balanced gut can positively influence the body's inflammatory response.

Add Herbs and Spices for Extra Benefits: Many herbs and spices contain compounds with anti-inflammatory properties. Regularly using ingredients like turmeric, ginger, and garlic not only enhances the flavor of your meals but also provides health benefits without adding extra calories.

Increase Fiber Intake: Fiber is essential for digestive health and can help lower inflammation levels. A diet rich in fiber supports a healthy gut microbiome, regulates blood sugar, and reduces the risk of chronic diseases. Include plenty of fruits, vegetables, whole grains, legumes, and seeds to meet your daily fiber needs.

Drink to Support Your Well-Being: Hydration plays a role in overall health and inflammation management. Choose water as your primary beverage, but also consider green tea, which contains antioxidants that may help reduce inflammation. Limit sugary drinks and excessive caffeine, which can contribute to inflammation.

Foods to Add

Fresh Fruits:
- Blueberries
- Strawberries
- Oranges
- Grapes (red and black)
- Cherries
- Apples
- Kiwi
- Pomegranate seeds
- Avocados
- Raspberries
- Pears
- Mango

Colorful Vegetables:
- Spinach
- Kale
- Broccoli
- Brussels sprouts
- Sweet potatoes
- Carrots
- Beets
- Red cabbage
- Zucchini
- Cauliflower
- Swiss chard
- Asparagus
- Cucumber

Healthy Fats:
- Extra virgin olive oil
- Avocados
- Chia seeds
- Flaxseeds
- Walnuts
- Almonds
- Hemp seeds
- Pumpkin seeds
- Pecans
- Sesame seeds
- Hazelnuts
- Macadamia nuts

Fatty Fish:
- Salmon
- Mackerel
- Sardines
- Herring
- Anchovies
- Trout
- Arctic char

Whole Grains:
- Quinoa
- Brown rice
- Oats (steel-cut or rolled)
- Buckwheat
- Barley
- Millet
- Farro
- Amaranth
- Wild rice

Legumes:
- Lentils
- Chickpeas
- Black beans
- Kidney beans
- Green peas
- Edamame
- Pinto beans
- White beans
- Fava beans

Herbs and Spices:
- Turmeric
- Ginger
- Garlic
- Cinnamon
- Basil
- Oregano
- Rosemary
- Thyme
- Sage
- Parsley
- Mint
- Cilantro

Fermented Foods:
- Sauerkraut (unpasteurized)
- Kimchi
- Kefir (unsweetened)
- Yogurt with live cultures
- Miso
- Tempeh
- Kombucha (low in sugar)
- Pickles (fermented, not vinegar-based)
- Natto

Green Tea and Herbal Teas:
- Green tea
- Matcha
- Ginger tea
- Peppermint tea
- Chamomile tea
- Rooibos tea
- Hibiscus tea
- Lemon balm tea

Lean Protein Sources:
- Skinless chicken breast
- Turkey
- Lean cuts of beef (sirloin, tenderloin)
- Rabbit meat
- Venison
- Bison
- Eggs (especially omega-3 enriched)

Chapter 2: Planning Your Anti-Inflammatory Journey

Setting Your Goals

Goals provide direction, motivation, and a sense of purpose, making it easier to stay committed to your new dietary and lifestyle choices. When setting your goals, keep the following principles in mind:

Be Specific

Your goals should be clear and specific to avoid ambiguity. Instead of a vague goal like "I want to be healthier," define what health improvement looks like for you. Are you aiming to reduce joint pain, lower your cholesterol levels, improve digestion, or boost your energy levels? For example, a specific goal could be, "I want to decrease my joint pain by following an anti-inflammatory diet rich in omega-3 fatty acids and antioxidants." The more detailed your goal, the easier it will be to create an action plan tailored to your needs.

Make Your Goals Measurable

Measurable goals enable you to track your progress and celebrate small victories along the way. If your goal is to reduce inflammation, consider using specific metrics such as monitoring the levels of inflammatory markers (like CRP) in your blood, tracking your weight, recording the frequency and intensity of flare-ups in chronic conditions, or even maintaining a symptom journal. Quantifying your progress helps you stay motivated and recognize the positive impact of your efforts.

Ensure Your Goals Are Achievable

While it's important to aim high and challenge yourself, your goals should also be realistic and attainable. Setting overly ambitious goals can lead to frustration and disappointment if they are not met. For example, instead of aiming to eliminate all inflammatory foods overnight, start with manageable steps like reducing processed sugar intake over the next two weeks. Assess your current lifestyle, resources, and health status to create goals that push you without overwhelming you.

Make Goals Relevant to Your Life

Your goals should align with your personal values, priorities, and life circumstances. Ask yourself why each goal matters to you. Is it to feel more energetic to keep up with your kids, to manage a chronic health condition, or to improve your overall quality of life? When your goals resonate with what truly matters to you, you're more likely to stay motivated and committed, even when faced with challenges. Personal relevance adds emotional weight, making your goals more meaningful and sustainable.

Set a Timeline

Setting a timeline for your goals creates urgency and keeps you focused. Deadlines promote consistent effort and help avoid procrastination. Consider both short-term goals, like trying an anti-inflammatory breakfast for two weeks, and long-term goals, such as maintaining the lifestyle for a year.

Here are some example goals you might consider when planning your wellness-focused lifestyle:

☐ **Reduce Inflammatory Markers:** Aim to lower the levels of inflammatory markers in your blood (such as C-reactive protein or IL-6) within a specific timeframe, as recommended by your healthcare provider.

☐ **Weight Management:** If weight is a concern, set a goal to achieve and maintain a healthy weight for your body type, which can reduce inflammation.

☐ **Improved Mobility:** If you have joint pain or stiffness, you might set a goal to improve your mobility, whether it's being able to walk a certain distance comfortably or perform specific exercises without discomfort.

☐ **Increase Energy Levels:** Many individuals notice an increase in energy when they follow an anti-inflammatory diet. Set a goal to have more energy for daily activities.

☐ **Manage a Specific Condition:** If you have a specific health condition affected by inflammation, such as rheumatoid arthritis, Crohn's disease, or psoriasis, work with your healthcare provider to establish condition-specific goals and track your progress.

☐ **Dietary Changes:** Consider setting goals related to dietary changes, such as increasing your daily intake of fruits and vegetables, reducing your intake of processed foods, or learning to cook anti-inflammatory recipes.

By setting clear and achievable goals that are tailored to your unique needs and aspirations, you'll give yourself a roadmap for your anti-inflammatory journey. These goals will guide your decisions and actions, making it easier to stay on course as you make important dietary and lifestyle changes.

Creating a Grocery List

A well-organized list will help you stock up on the foods you need while minimizing the temptation to buy items that don't align with your goals. Here's how to create an effective grocery list:

Plan Your Meals

Before you head to the store, take some time to plan your meals for the week. Think about what you'll eat for breakfast, lunch, dinner, and snacks. Consider your dietary restrictions, goals, and any specific recipes you want to try. Planning your meals will not only ensure you have the right ingredients but also save you time and money.

Ensure your grocery list includes a wide variety of anti-inflammatory foods, such as:

- ☑ **Fruits and Vegetables:** Choose a range of colorful fruits and vegetables to ensure you get a broad spectrum of vitamins, minerals, and antioxidants.

- ☑ **Fatty Fish:** Include fish like salmon, mackerel, and sardines, which are rich in omega-3 fatty acids.

- ☑ **Nuts and Seeds:** Add almonds, walnuts, chia seeds, and flaxseeds to your list.

- ☑ **Whole Grains:** Opt for whole grains like quinoa, brown rice, and whole wheat products.

- ☑ **Healthy Fats:** Don't forget extra virgin olive oil, which is a staple of the Mediterranean diet.

- ☑ **Herbs and Spices:** Include anti-inflammatory spices like turmeric, ginger, and cinnamon.

- ☑ **Lean Protein Sources:** Add lean protein sources like skinless poultry, beans, lentils, and tofu.

- ☑ **Probiotic Foods:** Consider yogurt, kefir, or sauerkraut to support a healthy gut.

Read Labels Carefully: When selecting packaged items, read labels to check for hidden inflammatory ingredients. Look out for high levels of added sugars, trans fats, and excessive sodium. Aim for products with a short ingredient list containing recognizable and whole ingredients.

Avoid Impulse Buying: Stick to your grocery list and avoid impulse buying, especially when it comes to unhealthy snacks or processed foods. If it's not on your list, take a moment to consider whether it aligns with your dietary goals before adding it to your cart.

Shop the Perimeter: In most grocery stores, the perimeter is where you'll find fresh produce, meat, and dairy sections, often containing the most anti-inflammatory foods. Try to focus your shopping on the perimeter and venture into the aisles only for specific items like whole grains, spices, or canned goods.

Buy in Bulk and Store Smartly: When it makes sense, consider buying items in bulk to save money. Be mindful of how you store your groceries. Proper storage can extend the shelf life of your fruits, vegetables, and other perishable items.

Use Technology: Consider using grocery list apps or digital note-taking tools to keep your list handy on your smartphone. Some apps even allow you to share your list with family members for collaborative shopping.

Here's a sample grocery list to help you get started with healthy, inflammation-reducing food choices:

- ☑ Fresh vegetables (e.g., spinach, broccoli, bell peppers, kale)
- ☑ Fresh fruits (e.g., blueberries, apples, oranges)
- ☑ Fatty fish (e.g., salmon)
- ☑ Nuts and seeds (e.g., almonds, chia seeds)
- ☑ Whole grains (e.g., quinoa, brown rice)
- ☑ Extra virgin olive oil
- ☑ Herbs and spices (e.g., turmeric, ginger, cinnamon)
- ☑ Lean protein sources (e.g., chicken breast, tofu)
- ☑ Probiotic-rich foods (e.g., yogurt)
- ☑ Canned tomatoes (low-sodium)
- ☑ Beans and lentils (e.g., black beans, green lentils)

By following these steps and maintaining an organized grocery list, you'll be better prepared to make healthy food choices and maintain a balanced, health-supporting diet with confidence.

Stocking Your Kitchen

Once you've set your goals and created a grocery list, the next step in your anti-inflammatory journey is to stock your kitchen with the essential ingredients and tools that will make your new lifestyle manageable and enjoyable. A well-prepared kitchen is the foundation for success. Here's how to get started:

Organize Your Kitchen Space: Begin by decluttering your kitchen. Remove expired or unhealthy items, freeing up space for your anti-inflammatory ingredients. A clean and organized kitchen makes meal preparation more efficient and enjoyable.

Essential Ingredients: Make sure you have a stock of essential anti-inflammatory ingredients. These may include fresh fruits and vegetables, whole grains, legumes, nuts, seeds, healthy oils like olive oil, and spices such as turmeric and ginger. Keeping these staples on hand will make it easier to prepare nutritious meals without last-minute grocery runs.

Food Storage Containers: Invest in good-quality food storage containers. Having a variety of sizes and shapes will make it easier to store leftovers and prepare meals in advance. Glass containers are preferable as they are more durable and do not leach harmful chemicals.

Kitchen Utensils: Ensure your kitchen is equipped with the necessary utensils and tools for meal preparation. These may include knives, cutting boards, measuring cups and spoons, mixing bowls, and a blender or food processor for smoothies and sauces.

Cookware and Bakeware: Use cookware made from safe materials such as stainless steel, cast iron, or non-toxic non-stick pans. Having a variety of pots, pans, and baking dishes will allow you to prepare a wide range of anti-inflammatory meals.

Food Labels and Reading Materials: Educate yourself on how to read food labels effectively. Familiarize yourself with terms like trans fats, added sugars, and sodium content. Having reference materials like recipe books or articles on anti-inflammatory eating can also be valuable for inspiration and guidance.

Meal Prep Tools: Consider investing in meal prep tools like a slow cooker, instant pot, or meal prep containers if you plan to prepare meals in advance. These can save you time and make it easier to stick to your diet.

Spacious Refrigerator and Freezer: Ensure your refrigerator and freezer are clean, spacious, and well-organized. Refrigerate perishable items like fresh produce and store frozen anti-inflammatory ingredients in the freezer for longer shelf life.

Water Filtration System: High-quality water is essential for your overall health. If your tap water quality is a concern, consider investing in a water filtration system to ensure you have access to clean, safe drinking water.

By stocking your kitchen with the right ingredients and tools, you'll set yourself up for a smooth transition to an anti-inflammatory diet. Your kitchen will become a hub for nutritious meals and a place where you can experiment with new recipes that support your journey to better health.

Meal Prep Tips

Planning and preparing your meals in advance not only saves you time and money but also ensures you have healthy options readily available, reducing the temptation to stray from your dietary goals. Here are some meal prep tips to help you get started:

Plan Your Meals in Advance

Planning is the foundation of successful meal preparation. Taking time each week to plan your meals not only reduces stress but also helps maintain consistency in following an anti-inflammatory diet. Consider what you'll eat for breakfast, lunch, dinner, and snacks. Make a detailed menu for the week and create a corresponding shopping list to ensure you have all the necessary ingredients on hand. This proactive approach minimizes last-minute unhealthy food choices.

Batch Cooking

Batch cooking involves preparing larger quantities of certain dishes and storing them for future meals. It's an efficient way to save time, reduce daily cooking stress, and ensure you always have healthy options available. Some batch-cooking ideas include:

- ☐ Cooking a big pot of whole grains like quinoa, brown rice, or farro to use throughout the week.

- ☐ Preparing a large batch of anti-inflammatory soup, stew, or chili and freezing individual portions for quick, nourishing meals.

- ☐ Roasting a tray of assorted vegetables, such as sweet potatoes, bell peppers, and broccoli, to incorporate into various dishes.

- ☐ Baking a batch of lean protein sources, such as chicken breast, turkey, or marinated tofu, to add to salads, wraps, or grain bowls.

Use Portion Control

One common pitfall in meal preparation is overeating. To avoid this, divide your batch-cooked dishes into individual portions immediately after cooking. Use portion control to help maintain a balanced diet, manage caloric intake, and support weight management goals. Consider using measuring cups, food scales, or portioned containers to maintain consistency.

Make Ahead Breakfasts

Prepare breakfast items in advance to streamline your morning routine, ensuring you start your day with a nutritious meal. Options like overnight oats with chia seeds, almond milk, and fresh berries; chia pudding topped with nuts and fruits; and frittatas filled with vegetables and lean proteins can be made the night before or in large batches. These breakfasts are easy to grab and packed with anti-inflammatory ingredients.

Organize Snacks

Having healthy snacks readily available helps prevent unhealthy impulse eating. Packaging snacks in portion-controlled containers makes it simple to grab a nutritious option when you're on the go. Consider anti-inflammatory snack choices such as:

- A small handful of raw nuts (almonds, walnuts) and seeds (pumpkin, sunflower).
- Greek yogurt with a sprinkle of flaxseeds or fresh fruit.
- Cut-up vegetables like carrots, cucumbers, and bell peppers paired with hummus or guacamole.

Pre-cut Fruits and Vegetables

Washing, cutting, and storing fruits and vegetables as soon as you get them home can save time during meal preparation. Having pre-cut produce ready to go encourages healthy snacking and makes it easier to throw together quick meals. Store them in clear containers to keep them visible and accessible.

Label and Date Items

When batch cooking and storing meals in the freezer, it's essential to label and date items clearly. This practice helps you easily identify the contents of each container, track how long items have been stored, and prevent food waste. Use freezer-safe labels or masking tape with a permanent marker to note the preparation date and dish name.

Schedule Prep Days

Designate one or two days a week as meal prep days. Use this time to cook, portion meals, and store them properly. Having a consistent schedule for meal prep can help establish a routine, making it easier to stick to your anti-inflammatory diet. Planning ahead reduces the temptation to opt for less healthy convenience foods during busy times.

Try Slow Cooker or Instant Pot Recipes

Slow cookers and Instant Pots are handy kitchen appliances, especially for busy individuals. They allow you to prepare healthy, flavorful meals with minimal effort. Consider exploring anti-inflammatory recipes designed for these devices, such as vegetable stews, lentil soups, or shredded chicken with anti-inflammatory spices like turmeric and ginger.

Stay Flexible

While planning is crucial, it's equally important to remain flexible. Life can be unpredictable, and there may be days when your meal plan needs to be adjusted. Be prepared to adapt by having a few versatile, quick-to-prepare ingredients on hand, like canned beans, frozen vegetables, or pre-cooked grains. Flexibility ensures you can continue making healthy choices even when your routine changes.

In the following chapters of this book, we'll delve deeper into the details of the 28-day meal plan and provide you with a variety of anti-inflammatory recipes for breakfast, lunch, dinner, and snacks to help you get started on your journey.

Chapter 3: The 28-Day Meal Plan

Day-by-Day Detox Meal Plan

Following a moderate-calorie anti-inflammatory diet can be beneficial for overall health. Excess body fat is associated with higher levels of inflammation, so a balanced approach to calorie intake may help reduce inflammatory markers. This meal plan prioritizes nutrient-dense, whole foods to support the body while minimizing inflammation.

Rather than a strict regimen, this plan serves as a flexible guideline adaptable to individual needs. Some recipes yield multiple servings, allowing portion adjustments based on hunger levels. Extra servings from lunch can also be used for dinner, making meal preparation easier and more efficient. If the calorie intake proves insufficient, additional recipes from the snacks section can be incorporated to meet energy requirements.

This plan provides a foundation for developing sustainable, anti-inflammatory eating habits tailored to individual preferences.

Week 1

Day 1	Monday
Breakfast (270 kcal)	Turmeric Scrambled Eggs. [p. 31]
A.M. Snack (200 kcal)	Apple Almond Dip - Slice 1 medium apple into wedges and dip into 1 tbsp almond butter.
Lunch (520 kcal)	Salmon Salad. [p. 45]
P.M. Snack (210 kcal)	Walnut Berry Mix - Measure 1/4 cup raw walnuts and eat with 1/2 cup fresh blueberries.
Dinner (400 kcal)	Turmeric Chickpea Curry. [p. 61]

Day 2	Tuesday
Breakfast (300 kcal)	Chia Seed Pudding. [p. 32]
A.M. Snack (190 kcal)	Cucumber Hummus Sticks - Cut 1 small cucumber and 1 medium carrot into sticks and dip into 3 tbsp hummus.
Lunch (470 kcal)	Quinoa and Black Bean Bowl. [p. 46]
P.M. Snack (180 kcal)	Chia Pear Slices - Slice 1 small pear into thin wedges and sprinkle with 1 tbsp chia seeds.
Dinner (380 kcal)	Baked Salmon with Asparagus. [p. 59]

Day 3	Wednesday
Breakfast (240 kcal)	Avocado Toast. [p. 33]
A.M. Snack (200 kcal)	Avocado Tomato Bites - Halve 1/2 cup cherry tomatoes and top each with 1 tsp mashed avocado.
Lunch (480 kcal)	Grilled Chicken and Quinoa Bowl. [p. 47]
P.M. Snack (220 kcal)	Almond Edamame Snack - Measure 1/2 cup shelled edamame and pair with 10 raw almonds.
Dinner (370 kcal)	Shrimp Cauliflower Rice Skillet. [p. 60]

Day 4	Thursday
Breakfast (280 kcal)	Oatmeal with Berries. [p. 34]
A.M. Snack (190 kcal)	Flax Berry Bowl - Measure 1/2 cup mixed berries and sprinkle with 1 tbsp ground flaxseeds and 1 tsp honey.
Lunch (370 kcal)	Mediterranean Tuna Wrap. [p. 48]
P.M. Snack (210 kcal)	Bell Pepper Guac Dip - Cut 1 medium bell pepper into strips and dip into 3 tbsp guacamole.
Dinner (370 kcal)	Grilled Vegetable and Quinoa Stuffed Peppers. [p. 62]

Day 5	Friday
Breakfast (250 kcal)	Greek Yogurt Parfait. [p. 35]
A.M. Snack (200 kcal)	Pumpkin Seed Celery - Spread 1 tbsp tahini on 2 celery stalks and sprinkle with 1 tbsp pumpkin seeds.
Lunch (430 kcal)	Crispy Bass with Citrus Soba. [p. 49]
P.M. Snack (190 kcal)	Kiwi Chia Scoop - Slice 1 medium kiwi in half, scoop out flesh, and top with 1 tbsp chia seeds.
Dinner (400 kcal)	Chopped Power Salad with Chicken. [p. 71]

Day 6	Saturday
Breakfast (270 kcal)	Quinoa Breakfast Bowl. [p. 36]
A.M. Snack (220 kcal)	Pecan Orange Slices - Peel 1 small orange, divide into segments, and pair with 1/4 cup pecans.
Lunch (420 kcal)	Chicken and Kale Caesar Salad. [p. 50]
P.M. Snack (210 kcal)	Carrot Almond Spread - Cut 2 medium carrots into sticks and dip into 1 tbsp almond butter.
Dinner (470 kcal)	Spiced Lentil and Vegetable Soup. [p. 65]

Day 7	Sunday
Breakfast (240 kcal)	Smoothie Bowl. [p. 37]
A.M. Snack (180 kcal)	Olive Tomato Mix - Halve 1/2 cup cherry tomatoes and toss with 10 pitted olives and 1 tsp olive oil.
Lunch (370 kcal)	Cauliflower Rice Bowl. [p. 51]
P.M. Snack (200 kcal)	Cashew Spinach Roll - Wrap 1/4 cup raw cashews in 2 large spinach leaves and eat as rolls.
Dinner (430 kcal)	Baked Spinach and Feta Pasta. [p. 66]

Week 2

Day 8	Monday
Breakfast (280 kcal)	Ginger-Tahini Buckwheat Pancakes. [p. 38]
A.M. Snack (200 kcal)	Apple Almond Dip - Slice 1 medium apple into wedges and dip into 1 tbsp almond butter.
Lunch (320 kcal)	Caprese Quinoa Salad. [p. 52]
P.M. Snack (210 kcal)	Walnut Berry Mix - Measure 1/4 cup raw walnuts and eat with 1/2 cup fresh blueberries.
Dinner (350 kcal)	Tofu and Vegetable Stir-Fry. [p. 67]

Day 9	Tuesday
Breakfast (220 kcal)	Sweet Potato Hash. [p. 39]
A.M. Snack (190 kcal)	Cucumber Hummus Sticks - Cut 1 small cucumber and 1 medium carrot into sticks and dip into 3 tbsp hummus.
Lunch (390 kcal)	Spicy Black Bean and Sweet Potato Bowl. [p. 53]
P.M. Snack (180 kcal)	Chia Pear Slices - Slice 1 small pear into thin wedges and sprinkle with 1 tbsp chia seeds.
Dinner (380 kcal)	Baked Eggplant with Tomato and Almond Topping. [p. 68]

Day 10	Wednesday
Breakfast (240 kcal)	Spinach and Mushroom Omelette. [p. 40]
A.M. Snack (200 kcal)	Avocado Tomato Bites - Halve 1/2 cup cherry tomatoes and top each with 1 tsp mashed avocado.
Lunch (460 kcal)	Zucchini Noodles with Pesto. [p. 54]
P.M. Snack (220 kcal)	Almond Edamame Snack - Measure 1/2 cup shelled edamame and pair with 10 raw almonds.
Dinner (350 kcal)	Grilled Shrimp and Pineapple Skewers. [p. 70]

Day 11	Thursday
Breakfast (240 kcal)	Berry Breakfast Quinoa. [p. 41]
A.M. Snack (190 kcal)	Flax Berry Bowl - Measure 1/2 cup mixed berries and sprinkle with 1 tbsp ground flaxseeds and 1 tsp honey.
Lunch (320 kcal)	Turkey and Avocado Lettuce Wraps. [p. 55]
P.M. Snack (210 kcal)	Bell Pepper Guac Dip - Cut 1 medium bell pepper into strips and dip into 3 tbsp guacamole.
Dinner (380 kcal)	Baked Eggplant with Tomato and Almond Topping. [p. 68]

Day 12	Friday
Breakfast (290 kcal)	Savory Quinoa Porridge. [p. 42]
A.M. Snack (200 kcal)	Pumpkin Seed Celery - Spread 1 tbsp tahini on 2 celery stalks and sprinkle with 1 tbsp pumpkin seeds.
Lunch (350 kcal)	Veggie Stir-Fry. [p. 56]
P.M. Snack (190 kcal)	Kiwi Chia Scoop - Slice 1 medium kiwi in half, scoop out flesh, and top with 1 tbsp chia seeds.
Dinner (370 kcal)	Spaghetti Squash with Pesto. [p. 69]

Day 13	Saturday
Breakfast (280 kcal)	Shakshuka with Spinach and Bell Peppers. [p. 43]
A.M. Snack (220 kcal)	Pecan Orange Slices - Peel 1 small orange, divide into segments, and pair with 1/4 cup pecans.
Lunch (490 kcal)	Baked Cod with Roasted Root Vegetables. [p. 57]
P.M. Snack (210 kcal)	Carrot Almond Spread - Cut 2 medium carrots into sticks and dip into 1 tbsp almond butter.
Dinner (380 kcal)	Eggs with Tomato, Chickpeas and Spinach. [p. 72]

Day 14	Sunday
Breakfast (270 kcal)	Buckwheat Porridge with Almond Butter and Fresh Figs. [p. 44]
A.M. Snack (180 kcal)	Olive Tomato Mix - Halve 1/2 cup cherry tomatoes and toss with 10 pitted olives and 1 tsp olive oil.
Lunch (440 kcal)	Mediterranean Grilled Fish with Spaghetti. [p. 58]
P.M. Snack (200 kcal)	Cashew Spinach Roll - Wrap 1/4 cup raw cashews in 2 large spinach leaves and eat as rolls.
Dinner (440 kcal)	Creamy Lemon-Spinach Spaghetti. [p. 63]

Week 3

Day 15	Monday
Breakfast (270 kcal)	Turmeric Scrambled Eggs. [p. 31]
A.M. Snack (200 kcal)	Apple Almond Dip - Slice 1 medium apple into wedges and dip into 1 tbsp almond butter.
Lunch (470 kcal)	Quinoa and Black Bean Bowl. [p. 46]
P.M. Snack (210 kcal)	Walnut Berry Mix - Measure 1/4 cup raw walnuts and eat with 1/2 cup fresh blueberries.
Dinner (380 kcal)	Baked Salmon with Asparagus. [p. 59]

Day 16	Tuesday
Breakfast (300 kcal)	Chia Seed Pudding. [p. 32]
A.M. Snack (190 kcal)	Cucumber Hummus Sticks - Cut 1 small cucumber and 1 medium carrot into sticks and dip into 3 tbsp hummus.
Lunch (480 kcal)	Grilled Chicken and Quinoa Bowl. [p. 47]
P.M. Snack (180 kcal)	Chia Pear Slices - Slice 1 small pear into thin wedges and sprinkle with 1 tbsp chia seeds.
Dinner (370 kcal)	Shrimp Cauliflower Rice Skillet. [p. 60]

Day 17	Wednesday
Breakfast (240 kcal)	Avocado Toast. [p. 33]
A.M. Snack (200 kcal)	Avocado Tomato Bites - Halve 1/2 cup cherry tomatoes and top each with 1 tsp mashed avocado.
Lunch (370 kcal)	Mediterranean Tuna Wrap. [p. 48]
P.M. Snack (220 kcal)	Almond Edamame Snack - Measure 1/2 cup shelled edamame and pair with 10 raw almonds.
Dinner (400 kcal)	Turmeric Chickpea Curry. [p. 61]

Day 18	Thursday
Breakfast (280 kcal)	Oatmeal with Berries. [p. 34]
A.M. Snack (190 kcal)	Flax Berry Bowl - Measure 1/2 cup mixed berries and sprinkle with 1 tbsp ground flaxseeds and 1 tsp honey.
Lunch (430 kcal)	Crispy Bass with Citrus Soba. [p. 49]
P.M. Snack (210 kcal)	Bell Pepper Guac Dip - Cut 1 medium bell pepper into strips and dip into 3 tbsp guacamole.
Dinner (370 kcal)	Grilled Vegetable and Quinoa Stuffed Peppers. [p. 62]

Day 19	Friday
Breakfast (250 kcal)	Greek Yogurt Parfait. [p. 35]
A.M. Snack (200 kcal)	Pumpkin Seed Celery - Spread 1 tbsp tahini on 2 celery stalks and sprinkle with 1 tbsp pumpkin seeds.
Lunch (420 kcal)	Chicken and Kale Caesar Salad. [p. 50]
P.M. Snack (190 kcal)	Kiwi Chia Scoop - Slice 1 medium kiwi in half, scoop out flesh, and top with 1 tbsp chia seeds.
Dinner (300 kcal)	Lemon Herb Baked Chicken. [p. 64]

Day 20	Saturday
Breakfast (270 kcal)	Quinoa Breakfast Bowl. [p. 36]
A.M. Snack (220 kcal)	Pecan Orange Slices - Peel 1 small orange, divide into segments, and pair with 1/4 cup pecans.
Lunch (370 kcal)	Cauliflower Rice Bowl. [p. 51]
P.M. Snack (210 kcal)	Carrot Almond Spread - Cut 2 medium carrots into sticks and dip into 1 tbsp almond butter.
Dinner (470 kcal)	Spiced Lentil and Vegetable Soup. [p. 65]

Day 21	Sunday
Breakfast (240 kcal)	Smoothie Bowl. [p. 37]
A.M. Snack (180 kcal)	Olive Tomato Mix - Halve 1/2 cup cherry tomatoes and toss with 10 pitted olives and 1 tsp olive oil.
Lunch (520 kcal)	Salmon Salad. [p. 45]
P.M. Snack (200 kcal)	Cashew Spinach Roll - Wrap 1/4 cup raw cashews in 2 large spinach leaves and eat as rolls.
Dinner (430 kcal)	Baked Spinach and Feta Pasta. [p. 66]

Week 4

Day 22	Monday
Breakfast (280 kcal)	Ginger-Tahini Buckwheat Pancakes. [p. 38]
A.M. Snack (200 kcal)	Apple Almond Dip - Slice 1 medium apple into wedges and dip into 1 tbsp almond butter.
Lunch (320 kcal)	Caprese Quinoa Salad. [p. 52]
P.M. Snack (210 kcal)	Walnut Berry Mix - Measure 1/4 cup raw walnuts and eat with 1/2 cup fresh blueberries.
Dinner (350 kcal)	Tofu and Vegetable Stir-Fry. [p. 67]

Day 23	Tuesday
Breakfast (220 kcal)	Sweet Potato Hash. [p. 39]
A.M. Snack (190 kcal)	Cucumber Hummus Sticks - Cut 1 small cucumber and 1 medium carrot into sticks and dip into 3 tbsp hummus.
Lunch (390 kcal)	Spicy Black Bean and Sweet Potato Bowl. [p. 53]
P.M. Snack (180 kcal)	Chia Pear Slices - Slice 1 small pear into thin wedges and sprinkle with 1 tbsp chia seeds.
Dinner (300 kcal)	Lemon Herb Baked Chicken. [p. 64]

Day 24	Wednesday
Breakfast (240 kcal)	Spinach and Mushroom Omelette. [p. 40]
A.M. Snack (200 kcal)	Avocado Tomato Bites - Halve 1/2 cup cherry tomatoes and top each with 1 tsp mashed avocado.
Lunch (460 kcal)	Zucchini Noodles with Pesto. [p. 54]
P.M. Snack (220 kcal)	Almond Edamame Snack - Measure 1/2 cup shelled edamame and pair with 10 raw almonds.
Dinner (350 kcal)	Grilled Shrimp and Pineapple Skewers. [p. 70]

Day 25	Thursday
Breakfast (240 kcal)	Berry Breakfast Quinoa. [p. 41]
A.M. Snack (190 kcal)	Flax Berry Bowl - Measure 1/2 cup mixed berries and sprinkle with 1 tbsp ground flaxseeds and 1 tsp honey.
Lunch (320 kcal)	Turkey and Avocado Lettuce Wraps. [p. 55]
P.M. Snack (210 kcal)	Bell Pepper Guac Dip - Cut 1 medium bell pepper into strips and dip into 3 tbsp guacamole.
Dinner (370 kcal)	Spaghetti Squash with Pesto. [p. 69]

Day 26	Friday
Breakfast (290 kcal)	Savory Quinoa Porridge. [p. 42]
A.M. Snack (200 kcal)	Pumpkin Seed Celery - Spread 1 tbsp tahini on 2 celery stalks and sprinkle with 1 tbsp pumpkin seeds.
Lunch (350 kcal)	Veggie Stir-Fry. [p. 56]
P.M. Snack (190 kcal)	Kiwi Chia Scoop - Slice 1 medium kiwi in half, scoop out flesh, and top with 1 tbsp chia seeds.
Dinner (400 kcal)	Chopped Power Salad with Chicken. [p. 71]

Day 27	Saturday
Breakfast (280 kcal)	Shakshuka with Spinach and Bell Peppers. [p. 43]
A.M. Snack (220 kcal)	Pecan Orange Slices - Peel 1 small orange, divide into segments, and pair with 1/4 cup pecans.
Lunch (490 kcal)	Baked Cod with Roasted Root Vegetables. [p. 57]
P.M. Snack (210 kcal)	Carrot Almond Spread - Cut 2 medium carrots into sticks and dip into 1 tbsp almond butter.
Dinner (440 kcal)	Creamy Lemon-Spinach Spaghetti. [p. 63]

Day 28	Sunday
Breakfast (270 kcal)	Buckwheat Porridge with Almond Butter and Fresh Figs. [p. 44]
A.M. Snack (180 kcal)	Olive Tomato Mix - Halve 1/2 cup cherry tomatoes and toss with 10 pitted olives and 1 tsp olive oil.
Lunch (440 kcal)	Mediterranean Grilled Fish with Spaghetti. [p. 58]
P.M. Snack (200 kcal)	Cashew Spinach Roll - Wrap 1/4 cup raw cashews in 2 large spinach leaves and eat as rolls.
Dinner (380 kcal)	Eggs with Tomato, Chickpeas and Spinach. [p. 72]

Staying on Track: Week 5 and Beyond

Congratulations on completing your 28-day journey through this anti-inflammatory meal plan! By now, you've experienced the benefits of incorporating anti-inflammatory foods into your daily life. However, the end of the initial four weeks doesn't mean the end of your journey. To continue reaping the rewards of reduced inflammation and better health, here are some key principles to help you stay on track:

Gradual Adaptations: As you progress into the fifth week and beyond, focus on making anti-inflammatory eating a permanent part of your lifestyle. Continue to implement what you've learned about food choices, meal planning, and preparation. Don't feel the need to make drastic changes, but rather aim for steady and sustainable adjustments to your diet.

Diversify Your Meals: One of the keys to long-term success is variety. Continue exploring new anti-inflammatory recipes, ingredients, and cooking techniques. Diversifying your meals keeps your taste buds engaged and ensures you receive a wide range of nutrients from different sources.

Monitor and Adjust: Listen to your body and be attuned to how it reacts to various foods. If you discover specific foods trigger inflammation or discomfort, consider eliminating or reducing them from your diet. On the flip side, pay attention to foods that make you feel great and energized and include more of them.

Keep a Food Journal: Maintaining a food journal can be a valuable tool. Document your daily meals and how you feel after consuming them. Over time, patterns may emerge, allowing you to make more informed decisions about your diet.

Set New Goals: Once you've completed the 28-day meal plan, consider setting new dietary goals. These could involve fine-tuning your current eating habits, trying different anti-inflammatory foods, or exploring specific health and wellness objectives.

Seek Support: Share your journey with friends and family who can provide encouragement and accountability. Consider joining online communities or support groups focused on anti-inflammatory diets, where you can connect with others on similar paths.

Stay Informed: Stay up-to-date with the latest research and developments in the field of anti-inflammatory nutrition. This knowledge will empower you to make informed choices and refine your dietary plan as needed.

Celebrate Milestones: Recognize and celebrate your achievements. Whether it's shedding a few pounds, improving your skin, or experiencing increased energy, take time to appreciate the positive changes in your life.

Professional Guidance: If you have specific health concerns or conditions that could benefit from an anti-inflammatory diet, consider consulting a healthcare professional or registered dietitian. They can provide personalized guidance and support to meet your unique needs.

Make It a Lifestyle: Ultimately, the key to lasting success is to view anti-inflammatory eating as a lifestyle, not a temporary diet. It's about making choices that promote wellness, vitality, and longevity. With time and consistent effort, the benefits will continue to enhance your overall health and well-being.

Chapter 4: Delicious Anti-Inflammatory Recipes

Breakfast Recipes

Start your day with a delicious and nutritious anti-inflammatory breakfast. These recipes are designed to kickstart your morning with flavors that delight your taste buds and support your well-being.

Turmeric Scrambled Eggs

Breakfast

Cooking time:
7 minutes

Prep time:
5 minutes

Servings:
2

Ingredients:

- 4 large eggs
- 1/2 teaspoon ground turmeric
- 1/4 teaspoon black pepper
- 1 cup fresh baby spinach, chopped
- 1 tablespoon extra virgin olive oil
- 1/2 avocado, sliced or diced
- Salt to taste
- Chopped fresh herbs (such as cilantro or parsley) for garnish (optional)

Directions:

- In a bowl, crack the eggs and whisk them together until the yolks and whites are well combined.
- In a small dish, mix the ground turmeric and black pepper. This helps distribute the turmeric evenly in the eggs.
- Heat a non-stick skillet over medium-low heat and add the olive oil.
- Once the oil is hot, add the chopped spinach to the skillet. Sauté it for 2–3 minutes or until it's slightly wilted.
- Push the sautéed spinach to the sides of the skillet, creating a clear space in the center.
- Pour the whisked eggs into the center of the skillet. Sprinkle the turmeric and black pepper mixture evenly over the eggs.
- Gently scramble the eggs with a spatula, incorporating the sautéed spinach, turmeric, and black pepper. Cook until the eggs are just set but still slightly creamy.
- Season with salt to taste and give the scrambled eggs a final stir.
- Remove the skillet from the heat and transfer the scrambled eggs to two plates.
- Top each serving with 1/4 of the avocado (sliced or diced) for added healthy fats and flavor.
- Garnish with chopped fresh herbs if desired, which not only adds flavor but also extra anti-inflammatory benefits.

Nutritional Value (per serving):

- Calories: Approx. 270 kcal
- Protein: 13 g
- Fat: 22 g
- Carbohydrates: 4 g
- Fiber: 2.5 g
- Sugar: 0.5 g
- Sodium: 160 mg

Chia Seed Pudding

Breakfast

Cooking time:
0 minutes

Prep time: 7 minutes,
plus chilling time: 3–4 h

Servings:
2

Ingredients:

- 1/4 cup chia seeds
- 1 cup unsweetened almond milk (or any preferred milk)
- 1/2 teaspoon ground turmeric
- 1/4 teaspoon ground cinnamon
- 1 tablespoon honey or maple syrup (adjust to taste)
- 1/2 teaspoon pure vanilla extract
- 2 tablespoons almond butter
- Fresh berries and 2 tablespoons sliced almonds for topping

Nutritional Value (per serving):

- Calories: Approx. 300 kcal
- Protein: 7 g
- Fat: 19 g
- Carbohydrates: 25 g
- Fiber: 10 g
- Sugar: 8 g
- Sodium: 90 mg

Directions:

- In a mixing bowl, combine chia seeds, unsweetened almond milk, ground turmeric, ground cinnamon, honey or maple syrup, vanilla extract, and almond butter.
- Whisk the mixture thoroughly to ensure that the chia seeds and almond butter are well combined and not clumped together. Taste the mixture and adjust the sweetness to your preference by adding more honey or maple syrup if needed.
- Cover the bowl with plastic wrap or a lid and refrigerate for at least 3–4 hours, or overnight for best results. During this time, the chia seeds will absorb the liquid and thicken, creating a pudding-like consistency.
- After chilling, give the pudding a good stir to redistribute the chia seeds evenly.
- To serve, divide the chia seed pudding into two serving dishes or jars.
- Top each serving with fresh berries and 1 tablespoon of sliced almonds, or any other anti-inflammatory toppings of your choice.

Avocado Toast

Breakfast

Cooking time:
5 minutes

Prep time:
10 minutes

Servings:
4

Ingredients:

- 2 ripe avocados
- 4 slices of whole-grain bread
- 1 clove of garlic, peeled
- 1 tablespoon extra virgin olive oil
- 1 teaspoon ground turmeric
- 1/2 teaspoon ground black pepper
- 1/2 teaspoon sea salt
- 1/2 lemon, juiced
- Red pepper flakes for garnish (optional)
- Fresh basil leaves or microgreens for garnish (optional)

Nutritional Value (per serving):

- Calories: Approx. 240 kcal
- Protein: 4 g
- Fat: 15 g
- Carbohydrates: 25 g
- Fiber: 8 g
- Sugar: 2 g
- Sodium: 400 mg

Directions:

- Toast the whole-grain bread slices until they are golden brown and crispy.
- Cut the ripe avocados in half, remove the pits, and scoop the flesh into a bowl. Mash the avocado with a fork until it's creamy with a few chunks remaining.
- Take the peeled garlic clove and rub it on the toasted bread slices. This adds a subtle garlic flavor to the toast.
- Drizzle a little extra virgin olive oil on each piece of toast.
- Spread the mashed avocado evenly on top of the garlic-rubbed toast slices.
- In a small bowl, mix the ground turmeric, ground black pepper, sea salt, and fresh lemon juice.
- Drizzle the turmeric-lemon mixture over the avocado-topped toast.
- Optionally, garnish with a sprinkle of red pepper flakes for added flavor and a touch of heat.
- For a finishing touch, add some fresh basil leaves or microgreens for extra nutrients and color.

Oatmeal with Berries

Breakfast

Cooking time:
8 minutes

Prep time:
5 minutes

Servings:
2

Ingredients:

- 1 cup old-fashioned oats
- 2 cups unsweetened almond milk (or any preferred milk)
- 1/2 teaspoon ground cinnamon
- 1/2 teaspoon ground turmeric
- 1/4 teaspoon ground black pepper
- 1 cup mixed berries (such as blueberries, strawberries, and raspberries)
- 1 tablespoon honey or maple syrup (optional, adjust to taste)
- 1/4 cup chopped walnuts or almonds (optional, for garnish)

Nutritional Value (per serving):

- Calories: Approx. 280 kcal
- Protein: 5 g
- Fat: 6 g
- Carbohydrates: 35 g
- Fiber: 7 g
- Sugar: 6 g
- Sodium: 200 mg

Directions:

- In a medium saucepan, combine the old-fashioned oats, unsweetened almond milk, ground cinnamon, ground turmeric, and ground black pepper.
- Heat the mixture over medium heat and bring it to a boil. Once boiling, reduce the heat to low and simmer for about 7–8 minutes, stirring occasionally. The oats should become creamy and soft.
- While the oatmeal is cooking, wash and prepare the mixed berries.
- Once the oatmeal reaches your desired consistency, remove it from the heat.
- If desired, sweeten the oatmeal with honey or maple syrup, adjusting the sweetness to your taste. Stir to combine.
- Divide the cooked oatmeal into serving bowls.
- Top the oatmeal with the mixed berries.
- Optionally, garnish with chopped walnuts or almonds for added crunch and nutrition.

Greek Yogurt Parfait

Breakfast

Cooking time:
0 minutes

Prep time:
7 minutes

Servings:
2

Ingredients:

- 1 cup plain Greek yogurt (unsweetened)
- 1/2 cup fresh mixed berries (such as blueberries, strawberries, and raspberries)
- 2 tablespoons honey or maple syrup (optional, adjust to taste)
- 1/4 cup chopped walnuts or almonds
- 1/2 teaspoon ground cinnamon
- 1/2 teaspoon ground turmeric
- Fresh mint leaves for garnish (optional)

Nutritional Value (per serving):

- Calories: Approx. 250 kcal
- Protein: 14 g
- Fat: 10 g
- Carbohydrates: 27 g
- Fiber: 4 g
- Sugar: 17 g
- Sodium: 60 mg

Directions:

- In a bowl, mix the plain Greek yogurt with ground cinnamon and ground turmeric. Stir until the spices are evenly distributed throughout the yogurt. If desired, sweeten the yogurt with honey or maple syrup, adjusting the sweetness to your taste.
- In two serving glasses or bowls, start by layering a portion of the spiced Greek yogurt.
- Add a layer of fresh mixed berries on top of the yogurt.
- Continue layering by adding more yogurt, followed by another layer of berries.
- Top the parfait with a sprinkle of chopped walnuts or almonds for added crunch and healthy fats.
- Optionally, garnish with fresh mint leaves for a burst of fresh flavor.

Quinoa Breakfast Bowl

Breakfast

Cooking time:
15 minutes

Prep time:
10 minutes

Servings:
2

Ingredients:

- 1/2 cup quinoa (uncooked)
- 1 cup unsweetened almond milk (or any preferred milk)
- 1/2 teaspoon ground turmeric
- 1/4 teaspoon ground cinnamon
- 1/4 teaspoon ground black pepper
- 1/2 cup fresh berries (e.g., blueberries, strawberries, or raspberries)
- 1 ripe banana, sliced
- 2 tablespoons chopped walnuts or almonds
- 1 tablespoon honey or maple syrup (optional, adjust to taste)
- Fresh mint leaves for garnish (optional)

Nutritional Value (per serving):

- Calories: Approx. 270 kcal
- Protein: 7 g
- Fat: 8 g
- Carbohydrates: 52 g
- Fiber: 7 g
- Sugar: 14 g
- Sodium: 100 mg

Directions:

- Rinse the quinoa thoroughly under running water to remove any bitterness.
- In a saucepan, combine the quinoa, unsweetened almond milk, ground turmeric, ground cinnamon, and ground black pepper.
- Bring the mixture to a boil over medium-high heat, then reduce the heat to low, cover, and simmer for about 15 minutes or until the quinoa is cooked and the liquid is absorbed. Stir occasionally.
- While the quinoa is cooking, prepare the fresh berries and banana slices.
- Once the quinoa is ready, fluff it with a fork and let it cool for a few minutes.
- Optionally, sweeten the quinoa with honey or maple syrup, adjusting the sweetness to your taste.
- Divide the cooked quinoa into two serving bowls.
- Top with fresh berries and banana slices.
- Sprinkle with chopped walnuts or almonds for added texture and healthy fats.
- Optionally, garnish with fresh mint leaves for extra freshness.

Smoothie Bowl

Breakfast

Cooking time:
0 minutes

Prep time:
8 minutes

Servings:
2

Ingredients:

- 2 ripe bananas, frozen
- 1 cup fresh spinach leaves
- 1/2 cup frozen pineapple chunks
- 1/2 cup unsweetened almond milk (or any preferred milk)
- 1 teaspoon ground turmeric
- 1/2 teaspoon ground ginger
- 1 tablespoon chia seeds
- 1/4 cup fresh berries (such as blueberries, strawberries, or raspberries)
- 2 tablespoons unsweetened shredded coconut
- 2 tablespoons chopped nuts (e.g., almonds, walnuts, or pecans)
- Fresh mint leaves for garnish (optional)

Nutritional Value (per serving):

- Calories: Approx. 240 kcal
- Protein: 6 g
- Fat: 10 g
- Carbohydrates: 52 g
- Fiber: 11 g
- Sugar: 26 g
- Sodium: 180 mg

Directions:

- In a high-speed blender, combine the frozen bananas, fresh spinach, frozen pineapple, unsweetened almond milk, ground turmeric, and ground ginger.
- Blend the mixture until it's smooth and creamy. You may need to stop and scrape down the sides of the blender as needed to ensure all ingredients are well mixed.
- Once the smoothie base is ready, divide it into two serving bowls.
- Top each bowl with a tablespoon of chia seeds for added fiber and omega-3 fatty acids.
- Add fresh berries on top for extra antioxidants and flavor.
- Sprinkle each bowl with unsweetened shredded coconut for texture and a hint of sweetness.
- Finish by garnishing with chopped nuts for healthy fats and crunch.
- Optionally, add fresh mint leaves for a refreshing touch.

Ginger-Tahini Buckwheat Pancakes

Breakfast

Cooking time:
10 minutes

Prep time:
10 minutes

Servings:
2

Ingredients:

- 1/2 cup buckwheat flour
- 1 teaspoon baking powder
- 1/2 teaspoon ground ginger
- 1/4 teaspoon ground cinnamon
- 1 tablespoon tahini (sesame paste)
- 1 tablespoon honey or maple syrup
- 3/4 cup unsweetened almond milk (or any preferred milk)
- 1 tablespoon extra virgin olive oil
- 1/4 cup fresh blueberries (for topping)
- 1 tablespoon chopped walnuts (for topping)

Nutritional Value (per serving):

- Calories: Approx. 280 kcal
- Protein: 7 g
- Fat: 16 g
- Carbohydrates: 35 g
- Fiber: 5 g
- Sugar: 10 g
- Sodium: 150 mg

Directions:

- In a mixing bowl, combine buckwheat flour, baking powder, ground ginger, and ground cinnamon. Stir to mix the dry ingredients evenly.
- In a separate small bowl, whisk together tahini, honey or maple syrup, and almond milk until smooth and well combined.
- Pour the wet mixture into the dry ingredients and stir gently with a spatula until a smooth batter forms. Let the batter rest for 5 minutes to thicken slightly.
- Heat a non-stick skillet over medium heat and add the olive oil.
- Once the oil is hot, spoon about 1/4 cup of batter per pancake into the skillet (you should get about 4 small pancakes total). Cook for 2–3 minutes on one side, or until bubbles form on the surface and the edges look set.
- Flip the pancakes and cook for another 2–3 minutes, until golden brown and cooked through.
- Remove the pancakes from the skillet and divide them between two plates.
- Top each serving with fresh blueberries and chopped walnuts for added flavor and anti-inflammatory benefits.

Sweet Potato Hash

Breakfast

Cooking time:
20 minutes

Prep time:
15 minutes

Servings:
4

Ingredients:

- 2 large sweet potatoes, peeled and diced
- 1 red bell pepper, diced
- 1 onion, diced
- 2 cloves garlic, minced
- 2 tablespoons extra virgin olive oil
- 1 teaspoon ground turmeric
- 1/2 teaspoon ground cumin
- 1/2 teaspoon ground paprika
- Salt and black pepper to taste
- Fresh cilantro or parsley for garnish (optional)

Nutritional Value (per serving):

- Calories: Approx. 220 kcal
- Protein: 2 g
- Fat: 7 g
- Carbohydrates: 23 g
- Fiber: 4 g
- Sugar: 6 g
- Sodium: 170 mg

Directions:

- In a large skillet, heat the olive oil over medium-high heat.
- Add the diced sweet potatoes and cook for about 5 minutes, stirring occasionally, until they start to soften.
- Add the diced red bell pepper and onion to the skillet and continue to cook for another 5–7 minutes, or until the sweet potatoes are tender and everything is slightly caramelized.
- Stir in the minced garlic, ground turmeric, ground cumin, and ground paprika. Cook for an additional 2–3 minutes, allowing the spices to bloom and the garlic to become fragrant.
- Season with salt and black pepper to taste. Adjust the seasonings to your preference.
- Remove the sweet potato hash from the heat and transfer it to a serving dish.
- Garnish with fresh cilantro or parsley, if desired, for added freshness.

Spinach and Mushroom Omelette

Breakfast

Cooking time:
15 minutes

Prep time:
10 minutes

Servings:
2

Ingredients:

- 4 large eggs
- 1 cup fresh spinach, chopped
- 1 cup sliced mushrooms
- 1/2 onion, finely chopped
- 1 clove garlic, minced
- 1 tablespoon extra virgin olive oil
- 1/2 teaspoon ground turmeric
- 1/4 teaspoon ground black pepper
- Salt to taste
- Fresh herbs (such as parsley or chives) for garnish (optional)

Nutritional Value (per serving):

- Calories: Approx. 240 kcal
- Protein: 12 g
- Fat: 12 g
- Carbohydrates: 6 g
- Fiber: 2 g
- Sugar: 2 g
- Sodium: 230 mg

Directions:

- In a mixing bowl, crack the eggs and whisk them together until the yolks and whites are well combined. Set aside.
- Heat the extra virgin olive oil in a non-stick skillet over medium heat.
- Add the chopped onions and sauté for 2-3 minutes or until they become translucent.
- Add the sliced mushrooms and continue to sauté for an additional 3-4 minutes until they are tender and any liquid has evaporated.
- Stir in the minced garlic and cook for another 30 seconds until fragrant.
- Add the chopped spinach to the skillet and cook for about 2 minutes until it wilts.
- Sprinkle the vegetables with ground turmeric and ground black pepper. Stir to combine.
- Pour the whisked eggs over the cooked vegetables, ensuring they are evenly distributed in the skillet.
- Cook the omelette over medium-low heat for 3-4 minutes or until the edges start to set.
- Gently lift the edges of the omelette with a spatula and tilt the skillet to let any uncooked eggs flow to the edges.
- Once the omelette is mostly set but slightly runny on top, carefully fold it in half.
- Cook for another 1–2 minutes or until the omelette is fully cooked through but still moist inside.
- Season with salt to taste.
- Optionally, garnish with fresh herbs such as parsley or chives for extra flavor and a pop of color.

Berry Breakfast Quinoa

Breakfast

Cooking time:
20 minutes

Prep time:
7 minutes

Servings:
2

Ingredients:

- 1/2 cup quinoa
- 1 cup water
- 1 cup unsweetened almond milk (or any preferred milk)
- 1/2 teaspoon ground cinnamon
- 1/4 teaspoon ground turmeric
- 1/4 teaspoon ground black pepper
- 1 cup mixed berries (such as blueberries, strawberries, and raspberries)
- 1/4 cup chopped nuts (e.g., almonds, walnuts, or pecans)
- 1 tablespoon honey or maple syrup (optional, adjust to taste)

Nutritional Value (per serving):

- Calories: Approx. 240 kcal
- Protein: 7 g
- Fat: 7 g
- Carbohydrates: 42 g
- Fiber: 5 g
- Sugar: 9 g
- Sodium: 120 mg

Directions:

- Rinse the quinoa thoroughly under running water to remove any bitterness.
- In a saucepan, combine the quinoa, water, unsweetened almond milk, ground cinnamon, ground turmeric, and ground black pepper.
- Bring the mixture to a boil over medium-high heat. Once boiling, reduce the heat to low, cover, and simmer for about 15–20 minutes, or until the quinoa is cooked and the liquid is absorbed. Stir occasionally.
- While the quinoa is cooking, prepare the mixed berries and nuts.
- Once the quinoa is ready, fluff it with a fork and let it cool for a few minutes.
- Optionally, sweeten the quinoa with honey or maple syrup, adjusting the sweetness to your taste. Stir to combine.
- Divide the cooked quinoa into two serving bowls.
- Top with mixed berries for extra antioxidants and flavor.
- Sprinkle with chopped nuts for added texture and healthy fats.

Savory Quinoa Porridge

Breakfast

Cooking time:
7 minutes

Prep time:
10 minutes

Servings:
2

Ingredients:

- 1 cup cooked quinoa
- 1 cup unsweetened almond milk (or any plant-based milk)
- 1 cup fresh spinach, chopped
- 1/2 cup cherry tomatoes, halved
- 1/2 avocado, sliced
- 1 tablespoon olive oil
- 1 tablespoon pumpkin seeds
- 1/2 teaspoon ground turmeric
- 1/4 teaspoon ground black pepper
- 1/4 teaspoon sea salt (adjust to taste)
- Juice of 1/2 lemon

Directions:

- In a small saucepan, combine the cooked quinoa and almond milk.
- Heat over medium heat, stirring occasionally, until warmed through.
- Add turmeric, black pepper, and sea salt, stirring well to combine.
- Add the chopped spinach and cook for another 2 minutes until wilted.
- Remove from heat and squeeze in fresh lemon juice.
- Divide the porridge into two bowls.
- Top with cherry tomatoes, avocado slices, pumpkin seeds, and a drizzle of olive oil.

Nutritional Value (per serving):

- Calories: Approx. 290 kcal
- Protein: 9 g
- Fat: 15 g
- Carbohydrates: 25 g
- Fiber: 6 g
- Sugar: 3 g
- Sodium: 200 mg

Shakshuka with Spinach and Bell Peppers

Breakfast

Cooking time:
20 minutes

Prep time:
10 minutes

Servings:
2

Ingredients:

- 4 large eggs
- 1 tablespoon olive oil
- 1 small red bell pepper, diced
- 1 small yellow bell pepper, diced
- 1 cup fresh spinach, chopped
- 1 small onion, finely chopped
- 2 cloves garlic, minced
- 1 can (14 oz) diced tomatoes (no added salt)
- 1 teaspoon ground cumin
- 1/2 teaspoon smoked paprika
- 1/4 teaspoon chili flakes (optional)
- 1/4 teaspoon sea salt (adjust to taste)
- 1/4 teaspoon ground black pepper
- Fresh parsley for garnish (optional)

Directions:

- Heat the olive oil in a large skillet over medium heat.
- Add the chopped onion and cook until translucent, about 3 minutes.
- Stir in the garlic, bell peppers, cumin, smoked paprika, chili flakes, salt, and black pepper. Cook for another 5 minutes until the peppers are softened.
- Pour in the diced tomatoes and simmer for 5 minutes, allowing the sauce to thicken slightly.
- Add the chopped spinach and stir until wilted.
- Make four small wells in the sauce and crack an egg into each well.
- Cover the skillet with a lid and cook for 5–6 minutes, or until the egg whites are set but the yolks remain runny.
- Remove from heat, garnish with fresh parsley if desired, and serve warm.

Nutritional Value (per serving):

- Calories: Approx. 280 kcal
- Protein: 13 g
- Fat: 12 g
- Carbohydrates: 15 g
- Fiber: 4 g
- Sugar: 6 g
- Sodium: 300 mg

Buckwheat Porridge with Almond Butter and Fresh Figs

Breakfast

Cooking time:
15 minutes

Prep time:
7 minutes

Servings:
2

Ingredients:

- 1/2 cup raw buckwheat groats, rinsed
- 1 1/2 cups unsweetened almond milk (or any plant-based milk)
- 1 tablespoon almond butter
- 2 fresh figs, sliced
- 1 tablespoon chia seeds
- 1 tablespoon maple syrup (optional)
- 1/4 teaspoon ground cinnamon
- 1/4 teaspoon sea salt
- Crushed almonds for garnish (optional)

Nutritional Value (per serving):

- Calories: Approx. 270 kcal
- Protein: 8 g
- Fat: 12 g
- Carbohydrates: 30 g
- Fiber: 6 g
- Sugar: 7 g
- Sodium: 180 mg

Directions:

- In a small saucepan, combine the rinsed buckwheat groats, almond milk, cinnamon, and sea salt.
- Bring to a gentle boil over medium heat, then reduce the heat and simmer for 10–12 minutes, stirring occasionally, until the buckwheat is tender and the mixture has thickened.
- Remove from heat and stir in the almond butter and chia seeds until well combined.
- If desired, add maple syrup for a touch of sweetness.
- Divide the porridge into two bowls.
- Top with fresh fig slices and garnish with crushed almonds if desired.

Lunch Recipes

Lunch is the perfect time to refuel and energize your body with satisfying, anti-inflammatory meals. These recipes are not only packed with flavor but also loaded with nutrients to support your well-being.

Salmon Salad

Lunch

Cooking time:
10 minutes

Prep time:
15 minutes

Servings:
2

Ingredients:

- 2 salmon fillets (about 6 oz each)
- 1 tablespoon extra virgin olive oil
- 1/2 teaspoon ground turmeric
- Salt and black pepper to taste
- 4 cups mixed greens (e.g., spinach, arugula, or kale)
- 1/2 cucumber, sliced
- 1/2 red onion, thinly sliced
- 1/2 cup cherry tomatoes, halved
- 1/4 cup Kalamata olives, pitted
- 1/4 cup feta cheese, crumbled (optional)

For the dressing:

- 2 tablespoons extra virgin olive oil
- 1 tablespoon lemon juice
- 1 clove garlic, minced
- 1/2 teaspoon ground turmeric
- Salt and black pepper to taste

Nutritional Value (per serving):

- Calories: Approx. 520 kcal
- Protein: 30 g
- Fat: 22 g
- Carbohydrates: 14 g
- Fiber: 4 g
- Sugar: 6 g
- Sodium: 400 mg

Directions:

- Preheat the oven to 400°F (200°C).
- Place the salmon fillets on a baking sheet lined with parchment paper. Drizzle them with 1 tablespoon of extra virgin olive oil and sprinkle with ground turmeric, salt, and black pepper.
- Bake the salmon in the preheated oven for about 10 minutes or until it flakes easily with a fork. Cooking time may vary depending on the thickness of the fillets.
- While the salmon is baking, prepare the salad. In a large bowl, combine the mixed greens, sliced cucumber, red onion, cherry tomatoes, and Kalamata olives.
- In a small bowl, whisk together the dressing ingredients: 2 tablespoons extra virgin olive oil, 1 tablespoon lemon juice, minced garlic, ground turmeric, salt, and black pepper.
- Once the salmon is cooked, remove it from the oven and let it cool for a few minutes.
- Break the salmon fillets into large chunks with a fork.
- Add the salmon chunks to the salad.
- Drizzle the dressing over the salad and gently toss everything to combine.
- Optionally, top the salad with crumbled feta cheese for extra flavor.

Quinoa and Black Bean Bowl

Lunch

Cooking time:
20 minutes

Prep time:
15 minutes

Servings:
2

Ingredients:

- 1 cup quinoa
- 2 cups water
- 1 can (15 oz) black beans, drained and rinsed
- 1 cup corn kernels (fresh, frozen, or canned)
- 1 red bell pepper, diced
- 1/2 red onion, finely chopped
- 1/2 cup chopped fresh cilantro
- 1/4 cup lime juice
- 2 tablespoons extra virgin olive oil
- 1 teaspoon ground cumin
- 1/2 teaspoon ground turmeric
- Salt and black pepper to taste
- Avocado slices for garnish (optional)

Nutritional Value (per serving):

- Calories: Approx. 470 kcal
- Protein: 10 g
- Fat: 7 g
- Carbohydrates: 47 g
- Fiber: 7 g
- Sugar: 4 g
- Sodium: 150 mg

Directions:

- Rinse the quinoa thoroughly under running water to remove any bitterness.
- In a saucepan, combine the quinoa and water. Bring it to a boil, then reduce the heat to low, cover, and simmer for about 15 minutes or until the quinoa is cooked and the liquid is absorbed. Fluff with a fork and let it cool.
- In a large mixing bowl, combine the cooked quinoa, black beans, corn, red bell pepper, and red onion.
- In a separate small bowl, whisk together the lime juice, extra virgin olive oil, ground cumin, ground turmeric, salt, and black pepper.
- Pour the dressing over the quinoa mixture and toss to combine.
- Stir in the fresh cilantro for added flavor.
- Optionally, garnish the bowls with avocado slices for creaminess and extra nutrients.

Grilled Chicken and Quinoa Bowl

Lunch

Cooking time:
15 minutes

Prep time:
10 minutes

Servings:
2

Ingredients:

- 2 small chicken breasts (about 8 oz total)
- 2 tablespoons extra virgin olive oil
- 1 teaspoon ground paprika
- 1/2 cup dry quinoa
- 2 cups mixed vegetables (e.g., broccoli florets, diced red bell pepper)
- 1/2 medium avocado, sliced
- 2 tablespoons lemon juice
- 1 teaspoon dried oregano
- Salt and black pepper to taste

Nutritional Value (per serving):

- Calories: Approx. 480 kcal
- Protein: 35 g
- Fat: 25 g
- Carbohydrates: 30 g
- Fiber: 8 g
- Sugar: 4 g
- Sodium: 350 mg

Directions:

- Rinse the dry quinoa under cold water. In a small pot, bring 1 cup of water to a boil, add the quinoa, reduce heat to low, cover, and simmer for 12–15 minutes until the water is absorbed and the quinoa is fluffy. Set aside.
- While the quinoa cooks, preheat a grill pan or regular skillet over medium heat.
- Rub the chicken breasts with 2 tablespoons of extra virgin olive oil, then sprinkle evenly with ground paprika.
- Grill the chicken for 6–7 minutes on each side, or until fully cooked (internal temperature reaches 165°F/74°C). Let it rest for 2 minutes, then slice into strips.
- While the chicken cooks, lightly sauté the mixed vegetables (broccoli and red bell pepper) in the same pan or steam them for about 5 minutes until tender but still crisp.
- In a large serving bowl, combine 1 cup of the cooked quinoa (about half of what you cooked, reserve any extra for later), sautéed vegetables, and sliced chicken.
- Divide the mixture evenly between two plates or bowls.
- Top each portion with half of the avocado slices.
- Drizzle each portion with 1 tablespoon of lemon juice, sprinkle with 1/2 teaspoon of dried oregano, and season with salt and black pepper to taste.

Mediterranean Tuna Wrap

Lunch

Cooking time:
0 minutes

Prep time:
15 minutes

Servings:
4

Ingredients:

- 2 cans (5 oz each) of canned tuna in water, drained
- 1/2 cup diced cucumber
- 1/2 cup cherry tomatoes, halved
- 1/4 cup red onion, finely chopped
- 1/4 cup Kalamata olives, pitted and sliced
- 2 tablespoons extra virgin olive oil
- 2 tablespoons lemon juice
- 1 teaspoon ground turmeric
- 1/2 teaspoon ground cumin
- Salt and black pepper to taste
- 4 whole-grain or whole-wheat tortillas
- 1 cup fresh spinach leaves
- 1/4 cup crumbled feta cheese (optional)

Nutritional Value (per serving):

- Calories: Approx. 370 kcal
- Protein: 20 g
- Fat: 12 g
- Carbohydrates: 18 g
- Fiber: 4 g
- Sugar: 3 g
- Sodium: 500 mg

Directions:

- In a large mixing bowl, combine the drained canned tuna, diced cucumber, cherry tomatoes, red onion, and Kalamata olives.
- In a separate small bowl, whisk together the extra virgin olive oil, lemon juice, ground turmeric, ground cumin, salt, and black pepper to create the dressing.
- Pour the dressing over the tuna and vegetable mixture and toss to combine.
- Warm the whole-grain or whole-wheat tortillas according to the package instructions.
- Lay out the warmed tortillas and divide the fresh spinach leaves evenly among them.
- Spoon the Mediterranean tuna mixture over the spinach leaves.
- Optionally, top each wrap with crumbled feta cheese for added creaminess and flavor.
- Roll up the tortillas, folding in the sides to create a wrap.

Crispy Bass with Citrus Soba

Lunch

Cooking time:
20 minutes

Prep time:
15 minutes

Servings:
2

Ingredients:

- 10 oz striped bass fillet (2 pieces, about 5 oz each)
- 4 oz 100% buckwheat soba noodles (dry)
- 1 cup snap peas, trimmed
- 2 tablespoons extra virgin olive oil
- 2 tablespoons fresh orange juice
- 1 teaspoon orange zest
- 1 teaspoon grated fresh ginger
- 1 clove garlic, minced
- 1 tablespoon chopped fresh cilantro (optional)
- Salt and black pepper to taste

Nutritional Value (per serving):

- Calories: Approx. 430 kcal
- Protein: 35 g
- Fat: 16 g
- Carbohydrates: 40 g
- Fiber: 5 g
- Sugar: 4 g
- Sodium: 300 mg

Directions:

- Cook soba noodles in boiling water according to package instructions (about 4–6 minutes), then drain and rinse under cold water. Set aside.
- Heat 1 tablespoon olive oil in a large nonstick skillet over medium heat. Season bass fillets with salt and pepper, then place skin-side down. Cook for 6–7 minutes until the skin is crispy and golden. Flip and cook for 2–3 minutes until opaque throughout. Remove and set aside.
- In the same skillet, add remaining 1 tablespoon olive oil. Sauté garlic and ginger for 1 minute until fragrant. Add snap peas and cook for 3–4 minutes until tender-crisp.
- Stir in orange juice, orange zest, and a pinch of salt. Add soba noodles and toss to coat, cooking for 2 minutes to heat through.
- Divide the soba and snap peas between two plates, top each with a bass fillet, and sprinkle with cilantro if using.

Chicken and Kale Caesar Salad

Lunch

Cooking time:
15 minutes

Prep time:
15 minutes

Servings:
2

Ingredients:

- 8 oz boneless, skinless chicken breast
- 2 tablespoons extra virgin olive oil
- 1 teaspoon garlic powder
- 4 cups chopped kale, stems removed
- 1/4 cup plain Greek yogurt
- 1 tablespoon lemon juice
- 1 teaspoon Dijon mustard
- 1 clove garlic, minced
- 1/2 cup whole-grain croutons
- Salt and black pepper to taste

Nutritional Value (per serving):

- Calories: Approx. 420 kcal
- Protein: 35 g
- Fat: 20 g
- Carbohydrates: 25 g
- Fiber: 5 g
- Sugar: 3 g
- Sodium: 400 mg

Directions:

- Heat 1 tablespoon of extra virgin olive oil in a large skillet over medium heat.
- Season the chicken breast with garlic powder, then add it to the skillet. Cook for 6–7 minutes on each side, or until fully cooked (internal temperature reaches 165°F/74°C). Let it rest for 2 minutes, then slice into strips.
- While the chicken cooks, prepare the dressing. In a small bowl, whisk together the Greek yogurt, lemon juice, Dijon mustard, minced garlic, and remaining 1 tablespoon of extra virgin olive oil until smooth.
- In a large bowl, massage the chopped kale with a few drops of lemon juice for 1–2 minutes to soften it slightly.
- Add the sliced chicken to the kale.
- Pour the dressing over the kale and chicken, and toss gently to coat evenly.
- Divide the salad evenly between two plates.
- Top each portion with 1/4 cup of whole-grain croutons.
- Season with salt and black pepper to taste, and serve immediately.

Cauliflower Rice Bowl

Lunch

Cooking time:
10 minutes

Prep time:
20 minutes

Servings:
4

Ingredients:

For the Cauliflower Rice:

- 1 large head of cauliflower, cut into florets
- 2 tablespoons extra virgin olive oil
- 1/2 teaspoon ground turmeric
- 1/2 teaspoon ground cumin
- 1/2 teaspoon ground paprika
- Salt and black pepper to taste

For the Toppings:

- 2 cups cooked chickpeas (canned or cooked from dry)
- 2 cups mixed greens (e.g., arugula, spinach, or kale)
- 1 red bell pepper, diced
- 1 cucumber, diced
- 1/4 cup pomegranate seeds
- 1/4 cup toasted pine nuts
- 1/4 cup chopped fresh cilantro

For the dressing:

- 3 tablespoons extra virgin olive oil
- 2 tablespoons lemon juice
- 1 clove garlic, minced
- Salt and black pepper to taste

Directions:

- **For the Cauliflower Rice:** Place the cauliflower florets in a food processor and pulse until they resemble rice or couscous.
- In a large skillet, heat the extra virgin olive oil over medium-high heat.
- Add the cauliflower rice and cook for 7–10 minutes, or until it's tender and slightly golden, stirring occasionally.
- Season the cauliflower rice with ground turmeric, ground cumin, ground paprika, salt, and black pepper. Stir to combine.
- **For the Toppings and Dressing:** In a large bowl, combine the cooked chickpeas, mixed greens, diced red bell pepper, diced cucumber, pomegranate seeds, and toasted pine nuts.
- In a small bowl, whisk together the dressing ingredients: extra virgin olive oil, lemon juice, minced garlic, salt, and black pepper.
- **To Serve:** Divide the spiced cauliflower rice among serving bowls.
- Top the cauliflower rice with the chickpea and vegetable mixture.
- Drizzle the dressing over the bowl.
- Garnish with chopped fresh cilantro.

Nutritional Value (per serving):

- Calories: Approx. 370 kcal
- Protein: 10 g
- Fat: 18 g
- Carbohydrates: 38 g
- Fiber: 12 g
- Sugar: 10 g
- Sodium: 450 mg

Caprese Quinoa Salad

Lunch

Cooking time:
15 minutes

Prep time:
15 minutes

Servings:
4

Ingredients:

- 1 cup quinoa
- 2 cups water
- 2 cups cherry tomatoes, halved
- 1 1/2 cups fresh mozzarella balls (mini bocconcini)
- 1/4 cup fresh basil leaves, torn
- 2 tablespoons extra virgin olive oil
- 1 tablespoon balsamic vinegar
- 1 clove garlic, minced
- Salt and black pepper to taste
- Optional: 1/4 cup pine nuts, toasted

Nutritional Value (per serving):

- Calories: Approx. 320 kcal
- Protein: 11 g
- Fat: 17 g
- Carbohydrates: 26 g
- Fiber: 3 g
- Sugar: 2 g
- Sodium: 200 mg

Directions:

- Rinse the quinoa thoroughly under running water to remove any bitterness.
- In a saucepan, combine the quinoa and water. Bring it to a boil, then reduce the heat to low, cover, and simmer for about 15 minutes or until the quinoa is cooked and the liquid is absorbed. Fluff with a fork and let it cool.
- In a large mixing bowl, combine the cooked quinoa, halved cherry tomatoes, fresh mozzarella balls, and torn fresh basil leaves.
- In a separate small bowl, whisk together the extra virgin olive oil, balsamic vinegar, minced garlic, salt, and black pepper to create the dressing.
- Drizzle the dressing over the quinoa mixture and toss to combine.
- Optionally, top the salad with toasted pine nuts for added texture and healthy fats.

Spicy Black Bean and Sweet Potato Bowl

Lunch

Cooking time:
25 minutes

Prep time:
15 minutes

Servings:
2

Ingredients:

- 1 medium sweet potato, peeled and diced (about 2 cups)
- 1 tablespoon extra virgin olive oil
- 1 teaspoon chili powder
- 1/2 teaspoon ground cumin
- 1 cup canned black beans, rinsed and drained
- 1/2 cup cooked brown rice
- 1/2 medium avocado, sliced
- 1/4 cup fresh salsa
- 1/4 cup chopped fresh cilantro
- 1 tablespoon lime juice
- Salt and black pepper to taste

Nutritional Value (per serving):

- Calories: Approx. 390 kcal
- Protein: 15 g
- Fat: 20 g
- Carbohydrates: 75 g
- Fiber: 15 g
- Sugar: 8 g
- Sodium: 450 mg

Directions:

- Preheat the oven to 400°F (200°C).
- In a medium bowl, toss the diced sweet potato with 1 tablespoon of extra virgin olive oil, chili powder, and ground cumin until evenly coated.
- Spread the sweet potato pieces in a single layer on a baking sheet lined with parchment paper. Roast in the preheated oven for 20–25 minutes, flipping halfway through, until tender and slightly crispy.
- While the sweet potato roasts, heat the black beans in a small saucepan over medium heat for 3–4 minutes, stirring occasionally, until warmed through. Alternatively, microwave them for 1–2 minutes.
- If not already prepared, warm the cooked brown rice in a microwave or on the stovetop with a splash of water for 1–2 minutes until heated through.
- In a large bowl, combine 1 cup of the roasted sweet potato, warmed black beans, and brown rice.
- Divide the mixture evenly between two serving bowls.
- Top each portion with half of the avocado slices and 2 tablespoons of fresh salsa.
- Sprinkle each bowl with 2 tablespoons of chopped cilantro and drizzle with 1/2 tablespoon of lime juice.
- Season with salt and black pepper to taste, and serve warm.

Zucchini Noodles with Pesto

 Lunch

 Cooking time:
0 minutes

 Prep time:
25 minutes

 Servings:
2

Ingredients:

For the Zucchini Noodles:

- 2 large zucchinis
- Salt to taste

For the Pesto:

- 2 cups fresh basil leaves
- 1/2 cup extra virgin olive oil
- 1/4 cup pine nuts, toasted
- 2 cloves garlic, minced
- 1/4 cup grated Parmesan cheese (optional)
- Juice of 1 lemon
- Salt and black pepper to taste

For Topping (optional):

- Cherry tomatoes, halved
- Extra pine nuts
- Fresh basil leaves
- Grated Parmesan cheese (optional)

Nutritional Value (per serving):

- Calories: Approx. 460 kcal
- Protein: 4 g
- Fat: 24 g
- Carbohydrates: 7 g
- Fiber: 2 g
- Sugar: 3 g
- Sodium: 200 mg

Directions:

- **For the Zucchini Noodles:** Using a spiralizer or a julienne peeler, create zucchini noodles from the two large zucchinis. If you prefer, you can also lightly steam the noodles for 1–2 minutes to soften them, but this is optional.
- Place the zucchini noodles in a colander, sprinkle with a little salt, and let them sit for about 15 minutes to release excess moisture. This will prevent your dish from becoming too watery.
- After 15 minutes, gently press the zucchini noodles between paper towels or a clean kitchen towel to remove the excess moisture.
- **For the Pesto:** In a food processor, combine the fresh basil leaves, extra virgin olive oil, toasted pine nuts, minced garlic, Parmesan cheese (if using), lemon juice, salt, and black pepper.
- Pulse until the mixture is well blended and has a pesto-like consistency.
- **To Assemble:** In a large bowl, toss the zucchini noodles with the prepared pesto sauce until they are well coated.
- Optionally, top the dish with halved cherry tomatoes, extra pine nuts, fresh basil leaves, and grated Parmesan cheese.

Turkey and Avocado Lettuce Wraps

Lunch

Cooking time:
10 minutes

Prep time:
15 minutes

Servings:
4

Ingredients:

- 1 pound ground turkey
- 1 tablespoon extra virgin olive oil
- 1 small onion, finely chopped
- 2 cloves garlic, minced
- 1 teaspoon ground turmeric
- 1/2 teaspoon ground cumin
- 1/2 teaspoon ground paprika
- Salt and black pepper to taste
- 1 ripe avocado, sliced
- 8 large lettuce leaves (e.g., iceberg or butter lettuce)
- 1/2 cup cherry tomatoes, halved
- Fresh cilantro leaves for garnish (optional)

Nutritional Value (per serving):

- Calories: Approx. 320 kcal
- Protein: 20 g
- Fat: 15 g
- Carbohydrates: 10 g
- Fiber: 4 g
- Sugar: 2 g
- Sodium: 200 mg

Directions:

- In a large skillet, heat the extra virgin olive oil over medium heat.
- Add the finely chopped onion and sauté for 2–3 minutes until it becomes translucent.
- Stir in the minced garlic and cook for an additional 30 seconds until fragrant.
- Add the ground turkey to the skillet and cook, breaking it into small pieces with a spatula, until it's browned and cooked through.
- Season the turkey with ground turmeric, ground cumin, ground paprika, salt, and black pepper. Stir to combine, and cook for an additional 2–3 minutes to infuse the flavors.
- While the turkey is cooking, prepare the avocado slices, lettuce leaves, and halved cherry tomatoes.
- Once the turkey mixture is ready, assemble the lettuce wraps. Place a spoonful of the turkey mixture onto each lettuce leaf.
- Top with avocado slices and halved cherry tomatoes.
- Optionally, garnish with fresh cilantro leaves for added flavor and freshness.

Veggie Stir-Fry

| Lunch | Cooking time: 15 minutes | Prep time: 15 minutes | Servings: 4 |

Ingredients:

For the Stir-Fry Sauce:

- 1/4 cup low-sodium soy sauce (or tamari for a gluten-free option)
- 2 tablespoons rice vinegar
- 1 tablespoon honey or maple syrup
- 1 teaspoon grated fresh ginger
- 1 clove garlic, minced
- 1/2 teaspoon ground turmeric
- 1/2 teaspoon ground cumin
- 1/4 teaspoon red pepper flakes (adjust to taste)

For the Stir-Fry:

- 2 tablespoons extra virgin olive oil
- 1 pound mixed vegetables (e.g., bell peppers, broccoli, snap peas, carrots, and mushrooms), sliced or chopped
- 1 cup tofu or tempeh, cubed (optional for added protein)
- 1 cup cooked quinoa or brown rice (for serving)
- Fresh cilantro or green onions for garnish (optional)
- Sesame seeds for garnish (optional)

Directions:

- **For the Stir-Fry Sauce:** In a small bowl, whisk together the low-sodium soy sauce (or tamari), rice vinegar, honey or maple syrup, grated fresh ginger, minced garlic, ground turmeric, ground cumin, and red pepper flakes. Set aside.
- **For the Stir-Fry:** Heat the extra virgin olive oil in a large skillet or wok over medium-high heat.
- Add the tofu or tempeh (if using) and sauté for a few minutes until it starts to brown. Remove from the skillet and set aside.
- In the same skillet, add the mixed vegetables and stir-fry for about 5–7 minutes until they are tender-crisp and slightly caramelized.
- Return the cooked tofu or tempeh to the skillet.
- Pour the prepared stir-fry sauce over the vegetables and tofu. Stir well to coat and heat through for an additional 2–3 minutes.
- Serve the veggie stir-fry over cooked quinoa or brown rice.
- Optionally, garnish with fresh cilantro, green onions, and sesame seeds.

Nutritional Value (per serving):

- Calories: Approx. 350 kcal
- Protein: 10 g
- Fat: 10 g
- Carbohydrates: 45 g
- Fiber: 7 g
- Sugar: 10 g
- Sodium: 700 mg

Baked Cod with Roasted Root Vegetables

Lunch

Cooking time:
35 minutes

Prep time:
15 minutes

Servings:
2

Ingredients:

- 2 cod fillets (about 6 oz each)
- 2 tablespoons extra virgin olive oil
- 1 teaspoon dried thyme
- 1 medium carrot, peeled and sliced (about 1 cup)
- 1 medium parsnip, peeled and sliced (about 1 cup)
- 1 small sweet potato, peeled and diced (about 1 cup)
- 1/2 cup diced red onion
- 1 tablespoon lemon juice
- 1/4 cup chopped fresh parsley
- Salt and black pepper to taste

Directions:

- Preheat the oven to 400°F (200°C).
- In a large bowl, toss the sliced carrot, parsnip, diced sweet potato, and red onion with 1 tablespoon of extra virgin olive oil and 1/2 teaspoon of dried thyme.
- Spread the vegetables in a single layer on a baking sheet lined with parchment paper. Roast in the preheated oven for 20 minutes.
- While the vegetables roast, rub the cod fillets with the remaining 1 tablespoon of extra virgin olive oil and sprinkle with the remaining 1/2 teaspoon of dried thyme.
- After 20 minutes, remove the baking sheet from the oven, push the vegetables to the sides, and place the cod fillets in the center.
- Drizzle the cod with 1 tablespoon of lemon juice.
- Return the baking sheet to the oven and bake for an additional 12–15 minutes, or until the cod flakes easily with a fork (internal temperature reaches 145°F/63°C) and the vegetables are tender.
- Remove from the oven and sprinkle the chopped parsley over the cod and vegetables.
- Divide the cod and roasted vegetables evenly between two plates.
- Season with salt and black pepper to taste, and serve warm.

Nutritional Value (per serving):

- Calories: Approx. 490 kcal
- Protein: 35 g
- Fat: 20 g
- Carbohydrates: 45 g
- Fiber: 8 g
- Sugar: 10 g
- Sodium: 350 mg

Mediterranean Grilled Fish with Spaghetti

Lunch

Cooking time:
20 minutes

Prep time:
20 minutes

Servings:
2

Ingredients:

- 10 oz white fish fillet (e.g., cod or tilapia, 2 pieces about 5 oz each)
- 6 oz whole wheat spaghetti (dry)
- 1 cup cherry tomatoes, halved
- 2 tablespoons extra virgin olive oil
- 1 tablespoon lemon juice
- 1 teaspoon dried oregano
- 1 clove garlic, minced
- 1 tablespoon chopped fresh parsley (optional)
- Salt and black pepper to taste

Nutritional Value (per serving):

- Calories: Approx. 440 kcal
- Protein: 32 g
- Fat: 16 g
- Carbohydrates: 45 g
- Fiber: 8 g
- Sugar: 4 g
- Sodium: 320 mg

Directions:

- Cook spaghetti in a pot of boiling salted water according to package instructions (about 10–12 minutes), then drain and set aside.
- Season fish fillets with 1 tablespoon olive oil, oregano, salt, and pepper. Heat a grill pan or skillet over medium heat and cook fish for 4–5 minutes per side until opaque and flaky.
- In a separate skillet, heat remaining 1 tablespoon olive oil over medium heat. Add minced garlic and sauté for 1 minute until fragrant.
- Add cherry tomatoes to the skillet and cook for 3–4 minutes until softened. Stir in lemon juice, salt, and pepper.
- Toss cooked spaghetti with the tomato mixture until well combined, cooking for an additional 2 minutes to heat through.
- Divide spaghetti between two plates, top each with a grilled fish fillet, and sprinkle with parsley if using.

Dinner Recipes

End your day with a satisfying and anti-inflammatory dinner. These recipes are not only flavorful but also packed with ingredients to help reduce inflammation and promote your overall health.

Baked Salmon with Asparagus

Dinner

Cooking time:
20 minutes

Prep time:
15 minutes

Servings:
4

Ingredients:

- 4 salmon fillets (about 6 oz each)
- 1 bunch of fresh asparagus, trimmed
- 2 tablespoons extra virgin olive oil
- 1 teaspoon ground turmeric
- 1/2 teaspoon ground cumin
- 1/2 teaspoon paprika
- Salt and black pepper to taste
- 1 lemon, thinly sliced
- Fresh dill or parsley for garnish (optional)

Nutritional Value (per serving):

- Calories: Approx. 380 kcal
- Protein: 30 g
- Fat: 18 g
- Carbohydrates: 7 g
- Fiber: 4 g
- Sugar: 3 g
- Sodium: 150 mg

Directions:

- Preheat your oven to 400°F (200°C).
- In a large mixing bowl, combine the trimmed asparagus with 1 tablespoon of extra virgin olive oil, ground turmeric, ground cumin, paprika, salt, and black pepper. Toss to coat the asparagus evenly with the seasoning.
- Place the salmon fillets on a baking sheet lined with parchment paper. Drizzle them with the remaining 1 tablespoon of extra virgin olive oil and season with salt and black pepper.
- Arrange the seasoned asparagus around the salmon on the baking sheet.
- Lay lemon slices on top of the salmon fillets.
- Bake in the preheated oven for about 15–20 minutes or until the salmon is cooked through, and the asparagus is tender.
- Optionally, garnish with fresh dill or parsley for added flavor.

Shrimp Cauliflower Rice Skillet

Dinner	Cooking time: 20 minutes	Prep time: 20 minutes	Servings: 2

Ingredients:

- 8 oz raw shrimp, peeled and deveined
- 3 cups cauliflower rice (from 1 small head, grated)
- 1 cup diced carrots
- 1/2 cup chopped green onions
- 1 clove garlic, minced
- 2 tablespoons extra virgin olive oil
- 1 tablespoon low-sodium soy sauce or tamari
- 1 teaspoon ground ginger
- Salt and black pepper to taste
- 1 tablespoon chopped fresh cilantro (optional)

Nutritional Value (per serving):

- Calories: Approx. 370 kcal
- Protein: 28 g
- Fat: 16 g
- Carbohydrates: 20 g
- Fiber: 6 g
- Sugar: 7 g
- Sodium: 600 mg

Directions:

- Heat 1 tablespoon olive oil in a large skillet over medium heat. Add shrimp, season with salt and pepper, and cook for 2–3 minutes per side until pink and opaque. Remove shrimp and set aside.
- In the same skillet, add remaining 1 tablespoon olive oil. Add garlic and sauté for 1 minute until fragrant.
- Add diced carrots and cook for 4–5 minutes until slightly softened, stirring occasionally.
- Stir in cauliflower rice and ground ginger, cooking for 5–7 minutes until the cauliflower softens and resembles fried rice.
- Add soy sauce or tamari, green onions, and cooked shrimp back to the skillet. Stir to combine and cook for 2 more minutes.
- Remove from heat, sprinkle with cilantro if using, and divide evenly between two plates.

Turmeric Chickpea Curry

Dinner

Cooking time:
25 minutes

Prep time:
15 minutes

Servings:
4

Ingredients:

- 2 tablespoons extra virgin olive oil
- 1 onion, finely chopped
- 2 cloves garlic, minced
- 1–inch piece of fresh ginger, minced
- 1 can (15 oz) chickpeas, drained and rinsed
- 2 cups canned or diced tomatoes
- 1 can (14 oz) coconut milk
- 1 tablespoon ground turmeric
- 1 teaspoon ground cumin
- 1 teaspoon ground coriander
- 1/2 teaspoon ground paprika
- Salt and black pepper to taste
- Fresh cilantro for garnish (optional)
- Cooked brown rice or quinoa for serving

Directions:

- In a large skillet or pot, heat the extra virgin olive oil over medium heat.
- Add the finely chopped onion and sauté for about 3–4 minutes until it becomes translucent.
- Stir in the minced garlic and ginger, and cook for an additional 30 seconds until fragrant.
- Add the ground turmeric, ground cumin, ground coriander, and ground paprika to the skillet. Stir to coat the onions and spices for 1–2 minutes.
- Add the canned chickpeas, diced tomatoes, and coconut milk to the skillet. Stir to combine.
- Season with salt and black pepper to taste. Bring the mixture to a boil, then reduce the heat to low and simmer for about 15–20 minutes, allowing the flavors to meld.
- Serve the turmeric chickpea curry over cooked brown rice or quinoa.
- Optionally, garnish with fresh cilantro for added flavor.

Nutritional Value (per serving):

- Calories: Approx. 400 kcal
- Protein: 10 g
- Fat: 23 g
- Carbohydrates: 30 g
- Fiber: 8 g
- Sugar: 6 g
- Sodium: 400 mg

Grilled Vegetable and Quinoa Stuffed Peppers

Dinner

Cooking time:
35 minutes

Prep time:
20 minutes

Servings:
4

Ingredients:

- 4 large bell peppers (any color)
- 1 cup quinoa, rinsed and drained
- 2 cups water or vegetable broth
- 2 cups mixed grilled vegetables (e.g., zucchini, eggplant, red onion, and bell peppers), chopped
- 1 can (15 oz) chickpeas, drained and rinsed
- 2 tablespoons extra virgin olive oil
- 1 teaspoon ground turmeric
- 1/2 teaspoon ground cumin
- 1/2 teaspoon ground paprika
- Salt and black pepper to taste
- Fresh basil or parsley leaves for garnish (optional)

Nutritional Value (per serving):

- Calories: Approx. 370 kcal
- Protein: 10 g
- Fat: 8 g
- Carbohydrates: 60 g
- Fiber: 11 g
- Sugar: 9 g
- Sodium: 300 mg

Directions:

- Preheat your grill to medium-high heat.
- While the grill is heating, cut the tops off the bell peppers and remove the seeds and membranes. Set aside.
- In a saucepan, combine the quinoa and water (or vegetable broth). Bring it to a boil, then reduce the heat to low, cover, and simmer for about 15 minutes or until the quinoa is cooked and the liquid is absorbed. Fluff with a fork and let it cool.
- Grill the mixed vegetables until they are tender and have grill marks, typically 5–7 minutes per side. Once done, remove from the grill and chop them.
- In a large mixing bowl, combine the cooked quinoa, grilled vegetables, chickpeas, extra virgin olive oil, ground turmeric, ground cumin, ground paprika, salt, and black pepper. Stir to combine.
- Preheat your oven to 375°F (190°C).
- Stuff each bell pepper with the quinoa and grilled vegetable mixture.
- Place the stuffed peppers in a baking dish, add about 1/4 inch of water to the bottom of the dish, and cover with foil.
- Bake in the preheated oven for about 20–25 minutes or until the peppers are tender.
- Optionally, garnish with fresh basil or parsley leaves for added flavor.

Creamy Lemon-Spinach Spaghetti

Dinner

Cooking time:
20 minutes

Prep time:
10 minutes

Servings:
2

Ingredients:

- 6 oz whole wheat spaghetti (dry)
- 3 cups fresh baby spinach
- 1/2 cup canned coconut milk (light)
- 2 tablespoons extra virgin olive oil
- 1 tablespoon lemon juice
- 1 teaspoon lemon zest
- 1 clove garlic, minced
- 1/2 teaspoon ground turmeric
- 2 tablespoons grated Parmesan (optional)
- Salt and black pepper to taste

Nutritional Value (per serving):

- Calories: Approx. 440 kcal
- Protein: 14 g
- Fat: 20 g
- Carbohydrates: 55 g
- Fiber: 8 g
- Sugar: 3 g
- Sodium: 350 mg

Directions:

- Cook spaghetti in a pot of boiling salted water according to package instructions (about 10–12 minutes), then drain and set aside.
- Heat 1 tablespoon olive oil in a large skillet over medium heat. Add minced garlic and sauté for 1 minute until fragrant.
- Stir in spinach and cook for 2–3 minutes until wilted.
- Add coconut milk, lemon juice, lemon zest, turmeric, salt, and pepper to the skillet. Simmer for 3–4 minutes, stirring occasionally, until the sauce thickens slightly.
- Toss cooked spaghetti into the sauce, mixing well to coat. Cook for an additional 2 minutes to heat through.
- Remove from heat, drizzle with remaining 1 tablespoon olive oil, and sprinkle with Parmesan if using.
- Divide evenly between two plates and serve warm.

Lemon Herb Baked Chicken

Dinner	Cooking time: 35 minutes	Prep time: 20 minutes	Servings: 4

Ingredients:

- 4 boneless, skinless chicken breasts
- 2 tablespoons extra virgin olive oil
- 1 lemon, zest and juice
- 2 cloves garlic, minced
- 1 teaspoon dried thyme
- 1 teaspoon dried rosemary
- 1/2 teaspoon ground turmeric
- Salt and black pepper to taste
- Fresh parsley for garnish (optional)

Nutritional Value (per serving):

- Calories: Approx. 300 kcal
- Protein: 30 g
- Fat: 11 g
- Carbohydrates: 5 g
- Fiber: 1 g
- Sugar: 1 g
- Sodium: 350 mg

Directions:

- Preheat your oven to 375°F (190°C).
- In a small bowl, combine the extra virgin olive oil, lemon zest, lemon juice, minced garlic, dried thyme, dried rosemary, ground turmeric, salt, and black pepper.
- Place the chicken breasts in a baking dish.
- Pour the lemon herb mixture over the chicken breasts and turn them to ensure they are well coated.
- Cover the baking dish and let the chicken marinate in the refrigerator for at least 15 minutes or up to an hour.
- After marinating, bake the chicken in the preheated oven for 30–40 minutes or until the chicken is cooked through and no longer pink in the center.
- Optionally, garnish with fresh parsley for added flavor.

Spiced Lentil and Vegetable Soup

Dinner

Cooking time:
25 minutes

Prep time:
15 minutes

Servings:
2

Ingredients:

- 1 cup dry green lentils
- 1 cup diced carrots
- 1 cup chopped zucchini
- 1/2 cup diced yellow onion
- 1 clove garlic, minced
- 2 cups vegetable broth
- 1/2 cup canned coconut milk
- 1 tablespoon extra virgin olive oil
- 1 teaspoon ground cumin
- 1/2 teaspoon ground turmeric
- 1/4 cup chopped fresh parsley
- Salt and black pepper to taste

Nutritional Value (per serving):

- Calories: Approx. 470 kcal
- Protein: 20 g
- Fat: 15 g
- Carbohydrates: 60 g
- Fiber: 15 g
- Sugar: 8 g
- Sodium: 450 mg

Directions:

- Rinse the dry green lentils under cold water until the water runs clear. Set aside.
- Heat 1 tablespoon of extra virgin olive oil in a medium pot over medium heat.
- Add the diced onion and sauté for 3–4 minutes, stirring occasionally, until softened and translucent.
- Stir in the minced garlic, ground cumin, and ground turmeric, and cook for 1 minute until fragrant.
- Add the diced carrots, chopped zucchini, rinsed lentils, and vegetable broth to the pot. Stir to combine.
- Bring the mixture to a boil, then reduce the heat to low, cover, and simmer for 20–25 minutes, or until the lentils and vegetables are tender.
- Stir in the coconut milk and cook for an additional 2 minutes to heat through.
- Remove from heat and stir in the chopped parsley.
- Divide the soup evenly between two bowls.
- Season with salt and black pepper to taste, and serve warm.

Baked Spinach and Feta Pasta

Dinner

Cooking time:
25 minutes

Prep time:
15 minutes

Servings:
2

Ingredients:

- 4 oz whole wheat penne pasta (dry)
- 3 cups fresh baby spinach
- 1/2 cup crumbled feta cheese
- 1 cup cherry tomatoes, halved
- 1 clove garlic, minced
- 2 tablespoons extra virgin olive oil
- 1 tablespoon lemon juice
- 1/2 teaspoon dried oregano
- Salt and black pepper to taste

Nutritional Value (per serving):

- Calories: Approx. 430 kcal
- Protein: 15 g
- Fat: 20 g
- Carbohydrates: 50 g
- Fiber: 8 g
- Sugar: 4 g
- Sodium: 450 mg

Directions:

- Preheat the oven to 375°F (190°C). Cook pasta in a pot of boiling salted water according to package instructions (about 10–12 minutes), then drain and set aside.
- In a large skillet, heat 1 tablespoon olive oil over medium heat. Add minced garlic and sauté for 1 minute until fragrant.
- Add cherry tomatoes and cook for 3–4 minutes until softened. Stir in spinach and cook for 2 minutes until wilted.
- In a large bowl, combine cooked pasta, spinach-tomato mixture, lemon juice, oregano, salt, and pepper. Toss to mix.
- Transfer the mixture to a small baking dish. Sprinkle crumbled feta cheese evenly over the top and drizzle with remaining 1 tablespoon olive oil.
- Bake for 10–12 minutes until the feta softens and slightly browns.
- Divide evenly between two plates and serve warm.

Tofu and Vegetable Stir-Fry

Dinner

Cooking time:
15 minutes

Prep time:
20 minutes

Servings:
4

Ingredients:

For the Stir-Fry Sauce:

- 1/4 cup low-sodium soy sauce (or tamari for a gluten-free option)
- 2 tablespoons rice vinegar
- 1 tablespoon honey or maple syrup
- 1 teaspoon grated fresh ginger
- 1 clove garlic, minced
- 1/2 teaspoon ground turmeric
- 1/2 teaspoon ground cumin
- 1/4 teaspoon red pepper flakes (adjust to taste)

For the Stir-Fry:

- 1 package (14 oz) extra-firm tofu, cubed
- 2 tablespoons extra virgin olive oil
- 1 red bell pepper, sliced
- 1 yellow bell pepper, sliced
- 1 small broccoli crown, cut into florets
- 1 carrot, thinly sliced
- 1 cup snap peas, trimmed
- Salt and black pepper to taste
- Cooked brown rice or quinoa for serving

Directions:

- **For the Stir-Fry Sauce:** In a small bowl, whisk together the low-sodium soy sauce (or tamari), rice vinegar, honey or maple syrup, grated fresh ginger, minced garlic, ground turmeric, ground cumin, and red pepper flakes. Set aside.
- **For the Stir-Fry:** Press the tofu to remove excess moisture, then cube it into bite-sized pieces.
- Heat 1 tablespoon of extra virgin olive oil in a large skillet or wok over medium-high heat.
- Add the cubed tofu and cook for 4–5 minutes, turning occasionally, until it's browned and slightly crispy. Remove the tofu from the skillet and set it aside.
- In the same skillet, add the remaining 1 tablespoon of extra virgin olive oil.
- Add the sliced red and yellow bell peppers, broccoli florets, sliced carrot, and snap peas to the skillet. Stir-fry for 5–7 minutes or until the vegetables are tender-crisp.
- Return the cooked tofu to the skillet.
- Pour the stir-fry sauce over the tofu and vegetables. Stir well to coat and heat through for an additional 2–3 minutes.
- Serve the tofu and vegetable stir-fry over cooked brown rice or quinoa.

Nutritional Value (per serving):

- Calories: Approx. 350 kcal
- Protein: 16 g
- Fat: 14 g
- Carbohydrates: 42 g
- Fiber: 9 g
- Sugar: 8 g
- Sodium: 600 mg

Baked Eggplant with Tomato and Almond Topping

Dinner

Cooking time:
35 minutes

Prep time:
20 minutes

Servings:
2

Ingredients:

- 1 medium eggplant (about 12 oz), sliced into 1/4–inch rounds
- 1 cup canned crushed tomatoes (no added sugar)
- 2 tablespoons extra virgin olive oil
- 1 clove garlic, minced
- 1 teaspoon dried oregano
- 1/4 cup almond flour
- 2 tablespoons nutritional yeast
- 1 tablespoon ground almonds (or finely chopped)
- 1 tablespoon fresh basil, chopped (optional)
- Salt and black pepper to taste

Nutritional Value (per serving):

- Calories: Approx. 380 kcal
- Protein: 12 g
- Fat: 25 g
- Carbohydrates: 30 g
- Fiber: 12 g
- Sugar: 10 g
- Sodium: 350 mg

Directions:

- Preheat the oven to 375°F (190°C). Line a baking sheet with parchment paper.
- Brush eggplant slices with 1 tablespoon olive oil, season with salt and pepper, and arrange in a single layer on the baking sheet. Bake for 15 minutes, flipping halfway, until softened.
- In a small skillet, heat remaining 1 tablespoon olive oil over medium heat. Add minced garlic and sauté for 1 minute until fragrant. Stir in crushed tomatoes, oregano, salt, and pepper. Simmer for 5–7 minutes until slightly thickened.
- In a small bowl, mix almond flour, nutritional yeast, ground almonds, and a pinch of salt to create a topping.
- Remove eggplant from the oven. Spoon tomato sauce over each slice, then sprinkle with the almond-yeast mixture.
- Return to the oven and bake for an additional 10–12 minutes until the topping is golden and crisp.
- Divide evenly between two plates, garnish with fresh basil if using, and serve warm.

Spaghetti Squash with Pesto

Dinner

Cooking time:
45 minutes

Prep time:
15 minutes

Servings:
4

Ingredients:

For the Spaghetti Squash:

- 2 medium spaghetti squashes
- 1 tablespoon extra virgin olive oil
- Salt and black pepper to taste

For the Pesto:

- 2 cups fresh basil leaves
- 1/2 cup extra virgin olive oil
- 1/4 cup pine nuts, toasted
- 2 cloves garlic, minced
- 1/4 cup grated Parmesan cheese (optional)
- Juice of 1 lemon
- Salt and black pepper to taste

For Topping (optional):

- Cherry tomatoes, halved
- Fresh basil leaves
- Grated Parmesan cheese (optional)

Nutritional Value (per serving):

- Calories: Approx. 370 kcal
- Protein: 5 g
- Fat: 27 g
- Carbohydrates: 15 g
- Fiber: 4 g
- Sugar: 5 g
- Sodium: 200 mg

Directions:

- **For the Spaghetti Squash:** Preheat your oven to 400°F (200°C).
- Cut the spaghetti squashes in half lengthwise and scoop out the seeds.
- Brush the cut sides of the squashes with extra virgin olive oil and season with salt and black pepper.
- Place the squash halves, cut side down, on a baking sheet lined with parchment paper.
- Roast in the preheated oven for about 30–45 minutes or until the squash is tender and the strands can be easily scraped with a fork.
- Let the squash cool for a few minutes, then use a fork to scrape the flesh into spaghetti-like strands.
- **For the Pesto:** In a food processor, combine the fresh basil leaves, extra virgin olive oil, toasted pine nuts, minced garlic, Parmesan cheese (if using), lemon juice, salt, and black pepper.
- Pulse until the mixture is well blended and has a pesto-like consistency.
- **To Assemble:** Toss the roasted spaghetti squash with the prepared pesto sauce until the strands are well coated.
- Optionally, top the dish with halved cherry tomatoes, fresh basil leaves, and grated Parmesan cheese.

Grilled Shrimp and Pineapple Skewers

Dinner

Cooking time:
10 minutes

Prep time:
15 minutes

Servings:
2

Ingredients:

- 8 oz raw shrimp, peeled and deveined
- 1 cup pineapple chunks (fresh or canned, drained)
- 1 cup diced red bell pepper
- 2 tablespoons extra virgin olive oil
- 1 tablespoon lime juice
- 1 teaspoon ground cumin
- 1/2 teaspoon smoked paprika
- 1/4 cup chopped fresh cilantro
- Salt and black pepper to taste

Nutritional Value (per serving):

- Calories: Approx. 350 kcal
- Protein: 25 g
- Fat: 20 g
- Carbohydrates: 35 g
- Fiber: 4 g
- Sugar: 20 g
- Sodium: 350 mg

Directions:

- Preheat a grill or grill pan to medium-high heat.
- In a medium bowl, toss the shrimp, pineapple chunks, and diced red bell pepper with 2 tablespoons of extra virgin olive oil, lime juice, ground cumin, and smoked paprika until evenly coated.
- Thread the shrimp, pineapple, and bell pepper alternately onto 4 skewers (metal or soaked wooden skewers).
- Grill the skewers for 2–3 minutes on each side, or until the shrimp are pink and opaque (internal temperature reaches 145°F/63°C) and the pineapple and peppers are lightly charred.
- Remove the skewers from the grill and sprinkle with chopped cilantro.
- Divide the skewers evenly between two plates (2 skewers per serving).
- Season with salt and black pepper to taste, and serve warm.

Chopped Power Salad with Chicken

Dinner	Cooking time: 20 minutes	Prep time: 15 minutes	Servings: 2

Ingredients:

- 8 oz boneless, skinless chicken breast
- 2 cups baby spinach, chopped
- 1 cup kale, chopped
- 1/2 cup shredded carrots
- 1/2 cup cucumber, diced
- 1/4 cup blueberries
- 2 tablespoons walnuts, chopped
- 1 tablespoon extra virgin olive oil (for cooking)
- 1 tablespoon extra virgin olive oil (for dressing)
- 1 tablespoon lemon juice
- 1 teaspoon Dijon mustard
- 1/2 teaspoon ground turmeric
- Salt and black pepper to taste

Directions:

- Season chicken breast with turmeric, salt, and pepper. Heat 1 tablespoon olive oil in a skillet over medium heat and cook chicken for 6–8 minutes per side until fully cooked. Let cool slightly, then chop into bite-sized pieces.
- In a large bowl, combine chopped spinach, kale, shredded carrots, diced cucumber, blueberries, and walnuts.
- In a small bowl, whisk together 1 tablespoon olive oil, lemon juice, Dijon mustard, salt, and pepper to make the dressing.
- Add chopped chicken to the salad mixture, drizzle with dressing, and toss to combine.
- Divide the salad evenly between two plates and serve immediately.

Nutritional Value (per serving):

- Calories: Approx. 400 kcal
- Protein: 30 g
- Fat: 22 g
- Carbohydrates: 15 g
- Fiber: 5 g
- Sugar: 6 g
- Sodium: 350 mg

Eggs with Tomato, Chickpeas and Spinach

Dinner

Cooking time:
20 minutes

Prep time:
10 minutes

Servings:
2

Ingredients:

- 4 large eggs
- 1 cup canned chickpeas, rinsed and drained
- 2 cups fresh spinach
- 1 cup canned crushed tomatoes
- 1 clove garlic, minced
- 1 tablespoon extra virgin olive oil
- 1/2 teaspoon ground cumin
- 1/4 teaspoon smoked paprika
- Salt and black pepper to taste
- 2 tablespoons chopped fresh cilantro (optional)

Nutritional Value (per serving):

- Calories: Approx. 380 kcal
- Protein: 20 g
- Fat: 18 g
- Carbohydrates: 30 g
- Fiber: 8 g
- Sugar: 6 g
- Sodium: 500 mg

Directions:

- Heat 1 tablespoon olive oil in a large skillet over medium heat. Add minced garlic and sauté for 1 minute until fragrant.
- Stir in crushed tomatoes, chickpeas, cumin, smoked paprika, salt, and pepper. Simmer for 5–7 minutes, stirring occasionally, until the sauce thickens slightly.
- Add spinach and cook for 2 minutes until wilted, stirring to combine with the sauce.
- Make 4 small wells in the sauce with a spoon. Crack an egg into each well.
- Cover the skillet and cook for 5–7 minutes, or until the egg whites are set but yolks remain runny (or cook longer if desired).
- Remove from heat, sprinkle with cilantro if using, and divide evenly between two plates.

Snack Recipes

Sometimes, you need a little something to keep you going during the day. These anti-inflammatory snack recipes are not only tasty but also loaded with ingredients that support your overall well-being.

Cucumber and Hummus

Snack

Cooking time:
0 minutes

Prep time:
10 minutes

Servings:
4

Ingredients:

- 2 large cucumbers, sliced into rounds or sticks
- 1 cup of your favorite hummus (store-bought or homemade)
- 1 tablespoon extra virgin olive oil
- 1/2 teaspoon ground turmeric
- Fresh parsley for garnish (optional)
- Salt and black pepper to taste

Directions:

- In a small bowl, combine the extra virgin olive oil and ground turmeric. Stir well to create a turmeric-infused olive oil.
- Arrange the cucumber slices or sticks on a serving platter.
- Drizzle the turmeric-infused olive oil over the cucumbers.
- Serve the cucumbers alongside a bowl of your favorite hummus.
- Optionally, garnish with fresh parsley for added flavor.

Nutritional Value (per serving):

- Calories: Approx. 180 kcal
- Protein: 8 g
- Fat: 13 g
- Carbohydrates: 16 g
- Fiber: 7 g
- Sugar: 2 g
- Sodium: 450 mg

Greek Yogurt and Berries

Snack

Cooking time:
0 minutes

Prep time:
5 minutes

Servings:
2

Ingredients:

- 1 cup Greek yogurt (plain, non-fat or low-fat)
- 1 cup mixed berries (e.g., blueberries, strawberries, raspberries)
- 1 tablespoon honey or maple syrup (optional)
- 1/2 teaspoon ground turmeric
- 1/2 teaspoon ground cinnamon
- Chopped nuts (e.g., almonds or walnuts) for garnish (optional)

Nutritional Value (per serving):

- Calories: Approx. 150 kcal
- Protein: 10 g
- Fat: 0 g
- Carbohydrates: 25 g
- Fiber: 4 g
- Sugar: 19 g
- Sodium: 50 mg

Directions:

- In a bowl, combine the Greek yogurt with ground turmeric and ground cinnamon. Stir well to mix the spices into the yogurt.
- Spoon the spiced Greek yogurt into serving bowls or glasses.
- Top the yogurt with a generous portion of mixed berries.
- If desired, drizzle honey or maple syrup over the berries for added sweetness.
- Optionally, garnish with chopped nuts for added texture and flavor.

Trail Mix

 Snack

 Cooking time:
0 minutes

 Prep time:
10 minutes

 Servings:
8

Ingredients:

- 1 cup raw almonds
- 1 cup raw walnuts
- 1/2 cup pumpkin seeds (pepitas)
- 1/2 cup dried tart cherries (unsweetened, if available)
- 1/2 cup dried blueberries (unsweetened, if available)
- 1/2 cup dark chocolate chips (at least 70% cocoa)
- 1 teaspoon ground turmeric
- 1/2 teaspoon ground cinnamon
- 1/4 teaspoon ground ginger
- Pinch of black pepper (to enhance turmeric absorption)
- Pinch of sea salt (optional)

Directions:

- In a large mixing bowl, combine the raw almonds, raw walnuts, pumpkin seeds, dried tart cherries, dried blueberries, and dark chocolate chips.
- In a small bowl, mix the ground turmeric, ground cinnamon, ground ginger, black pepper, and sea salt (if using).
- Sprinkle the spice mixture over the nut and fruit mixture.
- Use a large spoon to gently toss and mix the ingredients until the spices are evenly distributed.
- Store the anti-inflammatory trail mix in an airtight container or portion it into individual snack-sized bags for convenience.

Nutritional Value (per serving):

- Calories: Approx. 220 kcal
- Protein: 4 g
- Fat: 13 g
- Carbohydrates: 15 g
- Fiber: 3 g
- Sugar: 9 g
- Sodium: 30 mg

Carrot Sticks with Guacamole

Snack	Cooking time: 0 minutes	Prep time: 15 minutes	Servings: 4

Ingredients:

For the Guacamole:

- 2 ripe avocados, peeled and pitted
- 1 clove garlic, minced
- Juice of 1 lime
- 1/2 teaspoon ground turmeric
- 1/2 teaspoon ground cumin
- 1/2 teaspoon ground paprika
- Salt and black pepper to taste
- Fresh cilantro for garnish (optional)

For the Carrot Sticks:

- 4 large carrots, peeled and cut into sticks

Nutritional Value (per serving):

- Calories: Approx. 180 kcal
- Protein: 3 g
- Fat: 15 g
- Carbohydrates: 15 g
- Fiber: 9 g
- Sugar: 4 g
- Sodium: 150 mg

Directions:

- **For the Guacamole:** In a bowl, mash the ripe avocados with a fork until you reach your desired guacamole consistency (smooth or slightly chunky).
- Stir in the minced garlic, lime juice, ground turmeric, ground cumin, ground paprika, salt, and black pepper. Mix until all the ingredients are well combined.
- Optionally, garnish with fresh cilantro for added flavor.
- **For the Carrot Sticks:** Peel the carrots and cut them into sticks. You can make them as thin or thick as you prefer.
- Serve the carrot sticks alongside the guacamole for dipping.

Kale Chips

Snack

Cooking time:
20 minutes

Prep time:
10 minutes

Servings:
4

Ingredients:

- 1 bunch of fresh kale, preferably curly or Lacinato (dinosaur kale)
- 1 tablespoon extra virgin olive oil
- 1/2 teaspoon ground turmeric
- 1/2 teaspoon ground cumin
- 1/2 teaspoon paprika
- Salt and black pepper to taste

Nutritional Value (per serving):

- Calories: Approx. 70 kcal
- Protein: 2 g
- Fat: 4 g
- Carbohydrates: 5 g
- Fiber: 1 g
- Sugar: 0 g
- Sodium: 60 mg

Directions:

- Preheat your oven to 300°F (150°C).
- Wash the kale leaves and thoroughly dry them. Tear the leaves into bite-sized pieces, removing the tough stems.
- In a large bowl, drizzle the kale pieces with extra virgin olive oil.
- Sprinkle ground turmeric, ground cumin, paprika, salt, and black pepper over the kale.
- Toss the kale pieces well to ensure they are evenly coated with the oil and spices.
- Arrange the seasoned kale pieces in a single layer on a baking sheet lined with parchment paper.
- Bake in the preheated oven for about 20 minutes, or until the kale chips are crispy and have started to turn slightly brown. Keep a close eye on them to avoid burning.
- Remove the kale chips from the oven and let them cool for a few minutes.
- Serve your kale chips as a crunchy and nutritious snack.

Almonds and Dark Chocolate

Snack

Cooking time:
0 minutes

Prep time:
10 minutes

Servings:
6

Ingredients:

- 1 cup raw almonds
- 1/2 cup dark chocolate chips (at least 70% cocoa)
- 1/2 teaspoon ground turmeric
- 1/2 teaspoon ground cinnamon
- 1/4 teaspoon ground ginger
- A pinch of sea salt

Nutritional Value (per serving):

- Calories: Approx. 220 kcal
- Protein: 6 g
- Fat: 15 g
- Carbohydrates: 15 g
- Fiber: 4 g
- Sugar: 8 g
- Sodium: 30 mg

Directions:

- In a large mixing bowl, combine the raw almonds and dark chocolate chips.
- In a small bowl, mix the ground turmeric, ground cinnamon, ground ginger, and a pinch of sea salt.
- Sprinkle the spice mixture over the almonds and dark chocolate.
- Use a large spoon to gently toss and mix the ingredients until the spices are evenly distributed.
- Store the Almonds and Dark Chocolate mix in an airtight container or portion it into individual snack-sized bags for convenience.

Apple Slices with Almond Butter

Snack

Cooking time:
0 minutes

Prep time:
10 minutes

Servings:
4

Ingredients:

- 2 medium apples, cored and sliced into wedges
- 4 tablespoons almond butter (unsweetened)
- 1/2 teaspoon ground turmeric
- 1/2 teaspoon ground cinnamon
- 1/4 teaspoon ground ginger
- 1 teaspoon honey (optional, for drizzling)
- Chopped nuts (e.g., almonds or walnuts) for garnish (optional)

Nutritional Value (per serving):

- Calories: Approx. 180 kcal
- Protein: 7 g
- Fat: 18 g
- Carbohydrates: 30 g
- Fiber: 6 g
- Sugar: 20 g
- Sodium: 50 mg

Directions:

- In a small bowl, combine the almond butter, ground turmeric, ground cinnamon, and ground ginger. Mix well to create a spiced almond butter.
- Arrange the apple slices on a serving plate.
- Drizzle or spread the spiced almond butter over the apple slices.
- Optionally, drizzle honey over the almond butter for added sweetness.
- Garnish with chopped nuts if desired for added texture and flavor.

Peanut Butter Energy Balls

Snack

Cooking time:
0 minutes

Prep time:
15 minutes

Servings:
12 balls

Ingredients:

- 1 cup rolled oats (gluten-free if needed)
- 1/2 cup natural peanut butter (no added sugar or oils)
- 1/4 cup honey or maple syrup
- 2 tablespoons ground flaxseed
- 2 tablespoons chia seeds
- 1 teaspoon vanilla extract
- 1/2 teaspoon ground cinnamon
- Pinch of sea salt
- Optional: 1/4 cup chopped nuts (such as almonds, walnuts, or pecans)
- Optional: 1/4 cup dark chocolate chips (at least 70% cocoa)

Directions:

- In a large mixing bowl, combine rolled oats, peanut butter, honey or maple syrup, ground flaxseed, chia seeds, vanilla extract, cinnamon, and a pinch of sea salt. Mix well until all ingredients are evenly combined.
- If using, add chopped nuts and dark chocolate chips to the mixture and stir until distributed evenly.
- Once the mixture is well combined, place it in the refrigerator for about 15 minutes. Chilling will make it easier to roll into balls.
- After chilling, remove the mixture from the refrigerator. Take about a tablespoon-sized portion and roll it between your palms to form a ball. Repeat until all of the mixture is used, making Approx. 12 balls.
- Store the energy balls in an airtight container in the refrigerator for up to one week.

Nutritional Value (per serving):

- Calories: Approx. 120 kcal
- Protein: 4 g
- Fat: 7 g
- Carbohydrates: 11 g
- Fiber: 2 g
- Sugar: 5 g
- Sodium: 55 mg

Roasted Chickpeas

Snack

Cooking time:
40 minutes

Prep time:
10 minutes

Servings:
6

Ingredients:

- 2 cans (15 ounces each) chickpeas (garbanzo beans), drained and rinsed
- 2 tablespoons extra virgin olive oil
- 1/2 teaspoon ground turmeric
- 1/2 teaspoon ground cumin
- 1/2 teaspoon ground paprika
- 1/4 teaspoon cayenne pepper (adjust to taste)
- Salt and black pepper to taste

Nutritional Value (per serving):

- Calories: Approx. 180 kcal
- Protein: 7 g
- Fat: 7g
- Carbohydrates: 24 g
- Fiber: 6 g
- Sugar: 3 g
- Sodium: 300 mg

Directions:

- Preheat your oven to 400°F (200°C).
- Rinse and drain the chickpeas thoroughly. Pat them dry with a clean kitchen towel or paper towels to remove excess moisture.
- In a large bowl, combine the chickpeas with extra virgin olive oil, ground turmeric, ground cumin, ground paprika, cayenne pepper, salt, and black pepper. Toss well to ensure the chickpeas are evenly coated with the spices and oil.
- Spread the seasoned chickpeas in a single layer on a baking sheet lined with parchment paper.
- Roast in the preheated oven for about 40–45 minutes, or until the chickpeas are golden and crispy. Stir or shake the pan occasionally to ensure even roasting.
- Remove the roasted chickpeas from the oven and let them cool slightly before serving.

Sliced Bell Peppers with Salsa

Snack

Cooking time:
0 minutes

Prep time:
10 minutes

Servings:
4

Ingredients:

- 2 large bell peppers (red, yellow, or green), sliced into strips
- 1 cup homemade or store-bought salsa (look for a low-sodium option)
- 1/2 teaspoon ground turmeric
- 1/2 teaspoon ground cumin
- 1/2 teaspoon ground paprika
- Salt and black pepper to taste
- Fresh cilantro for garnish (optional)

Nutritional Value (per serving):

- Calories: Approx. 50 kcal
- Protein: 1 g
- Fat: 0 g
- Carbohydrates: 8 g
- Fiber: 2 g
- Sugar: 4 g
- Sodium: 250 mg (may vary depending on the salsa used)

Directions:

- Wash, core, and slice the bell peppers into strips. You can use a variety of colors for a more vibrant presentation.
- In a small bowl, combine the salsa with ground turmeric, ground cumin, ground paprika, salt, and black pepper. Stir well to create a spiced salsa.
- Arrange the bell pepper strips on a serving platter.
- Drizzle the spiced salsa over the bell peppers.
- Optionally, garnish with fresh cilantro for added flavor.

Chapter 5: Beyond the Diet

The Role of Exercise

Exercise and a healthy diet go hand-in-hand, offering a multitude of benefits, including mitigating inflammation. Incorporating regular physical activity into your lifestyle can significantly enhance the effects of an anti-inflammatory diet. Here's how exercise complements your anti-inflammatory efforts:

Reducing Inflammatory Markers

Regular physical activity has been shown to lower systemic inflammation by reducing the levels of certain inflammatory markers in the body, such as C-reactive protein (CRP) and interleukin-6 (IL-6). Exercise helps modulate the immune system, promoting a balanced response rather than an overactive inflammatory reaction. Both moderate aerobic exercise and strength training can contribute to this effect.

Weight Management

Exercise is a powerful tool for maintaining a healthy weight. Excess body fat, particularly around the abdomen, produces pro-inflammatory substances that can lead to chronic inflammation. By engaging in regular physical activity, you can burn calories, build lean muscle mass, and improve metabolism, all of which help reduce excess weight and, consequently, inflammation.

Improved Insulin Sensitivity

Regular exercise enhances insulin sensitivity, which helps regulate blood sugar levels and reduces the risk of developing type 2 diabetes. High insulin levels are associated with increased inflammation. Activities like brisk walking, cycling, and resistance training improve the body's ability to use insulin effectively, leading to lower blood sugar levels and a reduced inflammatory response.

Enhanced Blood Circulation

Exercise increases blood flow throughout the body, promoting the efficient delivery of oxygen and essential nutrients to tissues and the removal of metabolic waste products. Improved circulation supports the health of organs and tissues, reduces the risk of vascular inflammation, and aids in the recovery and repair processes.

Stress Reduction

Chronic stress triggers the release of cortisol, a hormone that can contribute to inflammation when elevated over long periods. Physical activity acts as a natural stress-reliever by stimulating the release of endorphins, the body's feel-good hormones. Mind-body exercises like yoga, tai chi, and even mindful walking can significantly lower stress levels, thus reducing stress-induced inflammation.

Joint Health

Engaging in activities that promote joint mobility and muscle strength, such as strength training, stretching, and low-impact exercises like swimming, can help alleviate pain and inflammation associated with conditions like arthritis. Regular movement helps maintain cartilage health, reduce stiffness, and support the muscles that stabilize joints, reducing the mechanical stress that can lead to inflammation.

Enhanced Antioxidant Defense

Exercise stimulates the body's natural antioxidant defense system. It increases the production of endogenous antioxidants, which help neutralize free radicals and reduce oxidative stress—one of the key contributors to chronic inflammation. Regular, moderate-intensity exercise can enhance this protective mechanism, supporting overall cellular health.

Improved Sleep

A regular exercise routine can improve sleep quality and duration, both of which are crucial for regulating inflammation. Physical activity helps synchronize your circadian rhythm, reduces symptoms of insomnia, and promotes deeper sleep stages. Quality sleep allows the body to repair and regenerate tissues, balance hormone levels, and reduce the production of pro-inflammatory cytokines.

Mood Regulation

Exercise has a positive impact on mental health and mood regulation, which is closely linked to inflammation levels. Physical activity helps alleviate symptoms of depression and anxiety by increasing the release of neurotransmitters like serotonin and dopamine. Better emotional well-being can lead to lower stress hormone levels, reducing stress-related inflammation and promoting overall health.

Incorporating a variety of exercises, such as aerobic activities, strength training, flexibility exercises, and mindfulness-based practices, can maximize these anti-inflammatory benefits. Aim for at least 150 minutes of moderate-intensity exercise per week, along with activities that support mobility, strength, and relaxation.

Managing Stress

Chronic stress can lead to a cascade of physiological responses that trigger inflammation, impacting your overall health. Incorporating stress management strategies into your daily life is an essential part of maintaining a healthy, balanced lifestyle. Here are some effective ways to manage stress:

Mindful Eating

Practice mindful eating to create a deeper connection between your mind and body. Focus on the present moment while eating, paying attention to the flavors, textures, and aromas of your food. Eat slowly, chew thoroughly, and savor each bite. This can enhance your appreciation of meals, improve digestion, and reduce stress associated with rushed or mindless eating.

Deep Breathing

Engage in deep breathing exercises to relax your mind and body. Deep breaths stimulate your body's relaxation response, lowering cortisol levels (the stress hormone) and reducing inflammation. Practice diaphragmatic breathing by inhaling deeply through your nose, allowing your abdomen to expand, holding for a few seconds, and exhaling slowly through your mouth. Aim to do this for 5–10 minutes daily.

Meditation and Yoga

Both meditation and yoga are powerful tools for stress reduction. Meditation helps calm the mind, improve focus, and foster a sense of inner peace. Yoga combines physical postures, breathing techniques, and meditation to reduce anxiety and enhance mental clarity. Regular practice can significantly lower stress levels and improve overall well-being.

Physical Activity

Regular exercise is not only anti-inflammatory but also an effective stress reliever. Activities such as walking, jogging, swimming, or dancing release endorphins, the body's natural mood elevators. Consistent physical activity helps reduce anxiety, improve sleep, and boost self-esteem, contributing to better stress management.

Adequate Sleep

Prioritize quality sleep to help your body recover from daily stressors. Aim for 7–9 hours of uninterrupted sleep per night. Establish a calming bedtime routine, avoid screens before bed, and create a sleep-friendly environment with a cool, dark, and quiet setting. Poor sleep can exacerbate stress and increase inflammation, so maintaining good sleep hygiene is crucial.

Time Management

Effective time management reduces the feeling of being overwhelmed. Break tasks into smaller, manageable steps, set realistic deadlines, and prioritize your responsibilities. Using tools like to-do lists, calendars, or time-blocking techniques can help you stay organized and reduce stress.

Seek Support

Connecting with others is vital for emotional well-being. Talk to trusted friends, family, or a mental health professional about your stressors. Sharing your thoughts and feelings can provide emotional relief, new perspectives, and practical solutions for managing stress.

Relaxation Techniques

Incorporate relaxation techniques such as progressive muscle relaxation, guided imagery, or mindfulness exercises into your daily routine. These practices can reduce physical tension, calm the nervous system, and promote a sense of relaxation and balance.

Laughter and Joy

Engage in activities that bring laughter and joy into your life. Watch a funny movie, play with pets, or spend time with people who make you smile. Laughter has been shown to decrease stress hormones, enhance mood, and support immune function.

Nature and Fresh Air

Spending time in nature and getting fresh air can be incredibly therapeutic. Activities like walking in a park, hiking, gardening, or simply sitting outdoors can help clear your mind, reduce stress, and improve your mood. Nature exposure also lowers cortisol levels and promotes relaxation.

Limit Stimulants

Be mindful of your intake of stimulants such as caffeine, nicotine, and sugary drinks, as they can heighten stress and anxiety for some individuals. Consider reducing or substituting these with herbal teas, water, or other calming beverages.

Creative Outlets

Engaging in creative activities provides a constructive outlet for stress. Whether it's painting, drawing, writing, playing a musical instrument, or crafting, creative expression can help process emotions, foster a sense of accomplishment, and bring joy.

Incorporating these stress management strategies into your routine can lead to improved mental, emotional, and physical health, supporting your overall well-being and reducing inflammation.

Quality Sleep

Poor sleep patterns can disrupt your body's natural processes, increase inflammation, and hinder your progress in adopting an anti-inflammatory lifestyle. Quality sleep is not just about the number of hours you get; it also involves the consistency, depth, and restorative nature of your rest. Here are some tips to help you improve the quality of your sleep:

Set a Consistent Sleep Schedule

Go to bed and wake up at the same time every day, even on weekends. This helps regulate your body's internal clock, also known as the circadian rhythm, making it easier to fall asleep and wake up naturally. Consistency helps improve sleep quality over time, leading to more restorative rest and better overall health.

Create a Relaxing Bedtime Routine

Engage in calming activities before bed, such as reading a book, taking a warm bath, listening to soothing music, or practicing relaxation exercises like deep breathing or meditation. Avoid stimulating activities like watching TV, using electronic devices, or engaging in stressful conversations, as these can increase alertness and delay sleep onset.

Make Your Sleep Environment Comfortable

Ensure your bedroom is conducive to sleep. Keep the room dark, quiet, and at a comfortable temperature (ideally between 60–67°F or 15–19°C). Use blackout curtains to block light, white noise machines to mask disruptive sounds, and invest in a comfortable mattress and pillows that support your preferred sleep position. A clutter-free, serene environment can also promote relaxation.

Limit Caffeine and Alcohol Intake

Caffeine and alcohol can disrupt sleep patterns, even if consumed hours before bedtime. Caffeine is a stimulant that can delay sleep onset, while alcohol may initially make you feel drowsy but can disrupt sleep cycles later in the night. Aim to avoid these substances at least 4–6 hours before bed.

Watch Your Diet

Avoid heavy, rich, or spicy meals close to bedtime. Large meals can cause discomfort and indigestion, making it harder to sleep. Opt for light, anti-inflammatory snacks if needed, such as a small handful of almonds, a banana, or a warm cup of herbal tea like chamomile, which can promote relaxation.

Limit Naps

While short power naps can be refreshing and boost productivity, long or irregular daytime napping can disrupt your sleep patterns. If you need to nap, keep it brief (20–30 minutes) and avoid napping late in the afternoon to prevent interference with your nighttime sleep.

Be Mindful of Your Screen Time

The blue light emitted by electronic devices can interfere with your sleep-wake cycle by suppressing melatonin production, a hormone that regulates sleep. Try to limit screen time in the evening, ideally for at least an hour before bed. Use "night mode" settings or blue light filters on your devices if evening use is necessary.

Keep a Sleep Diary

Consider keeping a sleep diary to track your sleep patterns, bedtime routines, and any factors that may affect your sleep quality. Record details such as bedtime, wake time, duration of sleep, quality of rest, and daily habits like caffeine intake, exercise, and stress levels. This can help you identify patterns and areas for improvement.

Manage Chronic Conditions

If you have a medical condition that affects your sleep, such as sleep apnea, chronic pain, restless leg syndrome, or acid reflux, seek appropriate treatment and guidance from a healthcare professional. Managing these conditions effectively can significantly improve your sleep quality.

Seek Professional Guidance

If you continue to struggle with sleep despite trying various strategies, consult with a healthcare professional or sleep specialist. There may be underlying issues, such as insomnia, sleep apnea, or other sleep disorders, that require medical evaluation and targeted treatment. Addressing these concerns can significantly enhance your sleep quality and overall well-being.

Adequate, high-quality sleep constitutes a fundamental pillar of an anti-inflammatory lifestyle. Prioritizing restorative sleep has been shown to play a crucial role in modulating inflammatory responses, thereby contributing to the reduction of systemic inflammation. Moreover, consistent, restful sleep supports optimal physiological functioning, cognitive performance, and emotional well-being.

Staying Hydrated

Dehydration can have detrimental effects on your body, potentially leading to increased inflammation. Here's why staying hydrated is crucial and some tips to help you maintain optimal hydration levels:

The Importance of Hydration

- **Cell Function:** Water is vital for the proper functioning of every cell in your body. It helps transport nutrients to cells and remove waste products.
- **Digestion:** Adequate hydration supports healthy digestion by facilitating the breakdown and absorption of nutrients.
- **Detoxification:** Water helps your body detoxify by flushing out toxins and waste materials through urine.
- **Body Temperature Regulation:** Proper hydration is necessary for maintaining a stable body temperature.
- **Joint Lubrication:** Hydration is essential for the lubrication of joints. Dehydration can contribute to joint pain and discomfort.
- **Skin Health:** Well-hydrated skin looks and feels better. Dehydrated skin may become dry, flaky, and prone to inflammation.

Tips for Staying Hydrated

- **Drink Water Regularly:** Make a conscious effort to sip water throughout the day, even if you don't feel thirsty. By the time you feel thirsty, you may already be mildly dehydrated.
- **Set Reminders:** Use alarms or reminders on your devices to prompt you to drink water at regular intervals.
- **Flavor with Fresh Ingredients:** Infuse your water with slices of citrus fruits, cucumber, mint leaves, or other fresh ingredients to make it more appealing.
- **Keep a Water Bottle Handy:** Carry a reusable water bottle with you wherever you go. Having it within arm's reach makes it more likely that you'll drink water regularly.
- **Monitor Your Urine Color:** A light, pale yellow color indicates proper hydration, while dark yellow or amber may be a sign of dehydration.
- **Drink Herbal Tea:** Herbal teas, like chamomile or ginger tea, can contribute to your daily fluid intake and provide additional anti-inflammatory benefits.
- **Choose Water-Rich Foods:** Many fruits and vegetables have high water content, such as watermelon, cucumbers, and oranges. Including these foods in your diet can help with hydration.
- **Adjust for Activity:** When you're more active or in hot weather, you may need to increase your water intake to compensate for fluid loss through sweat.
- **Limit Dehydrating Beverages:** Minimize the consumption of dehydrating beverages like sugary sodas, caffeinated drinks, and alcohol, which can contribute to fluid loss.
- **Listen to Your Body:** Pay attention to your body's signals. If you're feeling fatigued, experiencing headaches, or feeling thirsty, it may be a sign that you need to hydrate.

Tracking Your Progress

Tracking your journey helps you stay motivated, make informed decisions, and understand the impact of your efforts. Here are some methods and tips for tracking your progress:

Food Journal	Symptom Diary
Maintaining a food journal is an excellent way to record what you eat and how it makes you feel. Note the meals you consume, portion sizes, and any specific reactions or changes in symptoms you experience. This can help you identify foods that trigger inflammation or those that make you feel great.	If you have specific health concerns or symptoms related to inflammation, keep a symptom diary. Document the severity and frequency of your symptoms, as well as any patterns or triggers you notice. Over time, you may see improvements that indicate your anti-inflammatory efforts are working.

Monitoring your weight, body measurements, and body composition can provide insights into your progress. However, remember that improvements in your health and well-being go beyond just the numbers on a scale. Focus on how you feel and your overall health, not just your weight.

Lab Tests: If you have specific health conditions, consider regular check-ups and lab tests. These can measure inflammatory markers in your blood, such as C-reactive protein (CRP) or erythrocyte sedimentation rate (ESR). Improved results in these markers may indicate reduced inflammation.

Energy and Mood Levels: Pay attention to your energy levels and mood. Reduced fatigue and improved mood can be indicators of decreased inflammation. Note your overall sense of well-being.

Skin Health: Your skin can reflect changes in your diet and lifestyle. Document any improvements in skin conditions, such as clearer skin, reduced redness, or decreased inflammation-related skin issues.

Physical Performance: If you're engaging in regular exercise, track your physical performance. Are you able to complete workouts more easily, run farther, or lift more weight? These can be signs of reduced inflammation and improved fitness.

Consult with Professionals: Don't hesitate to consult with healthcare professionals or registered dietitians. They can provide guidance, perform assessments, and help you interpret your progress in the context of your specific health goals.

Before-and-After Photos: Taking before-and-after photos can provide a visual record of your progress. Sometimes, the changes in your appearance may be more apparent in photographs than on the scale.

Remember that everyone's journey is unique, and progress may vary from person to person. Stay patient and persistent, and use these tracking methods as tools to guide you on your anti-inflammatory path.

Chapter 6: Common Questions and Concerns

Dining Out While on an Anti-Inflammatory Diet

Eating at restaurants and social gatherings is an integral part of life, and maintaining your anti-inflammatory diet in such settings is entirely achievable. By adopting mindful strategies, you can make healthier choices without compromising the joy of dining out.

Plan Ahead: Prior to visiting a restaurant, take time to review the menu online if available. This enables you to identify dishes that align with your anti-inflammatory goals. Look for meals rich in vegetables, lean proteins, whole grains, and healthy fats. Additionally, reading customer reviews may provide insights into portion sizes and ingredient quality.

Communicate Your Needs: Effective communication with restaurant staff is key. Don't hesitate to express your dietary preferences clearly and politely. Inquire about ingredients, preparation methods, and potential modifications to ensure your meal meets your dietary needs. Many establishments are accommodating, especially when requests are made respectfully.

Choose Wisely: Select dishes that feature anti-inflammatory ingredients such as leafy greens, colorful vegetables, legumes, nuts, seeds, and fatty fish rich in omega-3s. Grilled, baked, steamed, or roasted items are preferable over fried or heavily processed foods. Prioritize simple, whole-food-based meals with minimal sauces and additives.

Watch Portions: Restaurant portions often exceed standard serving sizes. To manage this, consider sharing a dish with a dining companion or requesting a to-go container at the start of your meal to set aside half for later. This approach helps with portion control while reducing food waste.

Request Modifications: Feel empowered to customize your meal. Ask for dressings and sauces on the side, substitute refined grains with whole grains, and replace high-calorie sides with vegetables or salads. Such modifications can significantly reduce unhealthy fats, sugars, and sodium in your meal.

Be Mindful of Hidden Ingredients: Sauces, dressings, marinades, and condiments often contain hidden sugars, unhealthy fats, and sodium. Request ingredient details if unsure and opt for simple seasonings like olive oil, lemon, or vinegar to enhance flavor without compromising your diet.

Practice Portion Control: In addition to managing portion sizes through sharing or leftovers, eat slowly and attentively. Recognizing your body's hunger and satiety signals can prevent overeating and promote better digestion.

Be Careful with Drinks: Beverages can be hidden sources of sugars and empty calories. Avoid sugary cocktails, sodas, and excessive alcohol consumption, which can contribute to inflammation. Opt for water, sparkling water with lemon, herbal teas, or moderate amounts of red wine, which contains anti-inflammatory polyphenols.

Stay Hydrated: Drinking water throughout your meal aids digestion and helps regulate appetite. Sometimes, feelings of hunger are actually signs of dehydration. Starting with a glass of water before your meal can help manage portion sizes naturally.

Skip the Bread Basket: Bread baskets, often filled with refined carbohydrates, can lead to unnecessary calorie intake. Politely declining or asking the server not to bring bread to the table helps maintain your dietary discipline.

Practice Mindful Eating: Mindful eating fosters a healthier relationship with food. Focus on the sensory experience of eating—savor the flavors, textures, and aromas. This practice not only enhances enjoyment but also helps you recognize fullness cues, reducing the likelihood of overeating.

Dessert Alternatives: If you desire something sweet, choose healthier options like fresh fruit, sorbet, or a small serving of dark chocolate. These alternatives satisfy sweet cravings without excessive sugars and unhealthy fats.

Special Diets: For specific dietary needs or food allergies, inform the restaurant in advance. Many establishments can accommodate requests such as gluten-free, dairy-free, or vegan options, ensuring your meal aligns with your health requirements.

Enjoy the Social Aspect: Remember that dining out is not solely about food—it's an opportunity to connect with others. Focus on the social experience, engaging in meaningful conversations and enjoying the ambiance. This mindset reduces the stress of strict dietary adherence.

Be Flexible: While consistency is key to an anti-inflammatory lifestyle, occasional flexibility is natural. One indulgent meal won't negate your progress. Embrace balance, enjoy the experience, and return to your healthy routine with confidence.

With a little planning and mindfulness, dining out while following an anti-inflammatory diet can be an enjoyable experience. These strategies can help you make healthier choices and stay on track with your dietary goals, even when you're not in control of the kitchen.

Dealing with Food Allergies

If you have food allergies, following an anti-inflammatory diet can be more challenging, but it's entirely possible with the right strategies. Allergies to specific foods can cause inflammation and a range of symptoms, so it's crucial to be vigilant about what you eat. Here are some comprehensive tips for managing food allergies while maintaining an anti-inflammatory lifestyle:

Know Your Allergens: First and foremost, identify the foods to which you are allergic. Common allergens include nuts, shellfish, eggs, dairy, soy, and wheat, among others. It's important to recognize both obvious sources and hidden derivatives of these allergens in packaged and prepared foods. Keeping a food diary and working with an allergist can help pinpoint specific triggers.

Read Labels Carefully: When grocery shopping, meticulously read food labels to check for potential allergens. Look for any mentions of your allergens, including "may contain," "processed in a facility that also processes," or "shared equipment" statements. Familiarize yourself with alternative names for allergens, as they may appear under different terms on ingredient lists.

Communicate with Restaurants: When dining out, clearly communicate your allergies to restaurant staff. Inform your server about your specific allergies and ask detailed questions about the ingredients and preparation methods. Many restaurants offer allergen-specific menus or can make accommodations if you request in advance. Don't hesitate to speak directly with the chef if necessary.

Cook at Home: Preparing meals at home allows you to maintain complete control over the ingredients and cooking environment. This minimizes the risk of accidental exposure to allergens. Batch cooking and meal prepping can help save time while ensuring your meals are safe and aligned with your anti-inflammatory goals.

Substitute Ingredients: Get creative with ingredient substitutions to maintain variety in your diet. For example, use oat milk or coconut milk instead of dairy, and try quinoa flour or almond flour as gluten-free alternatives. There are numerous allergen-free products available that cater to specific dietary needs, helping you enjoy diverse and flavorful meals.

Avoid Cross-Contamination: Prevent cross-contamination in your kitchen by using separate utensils, cutting boards, and cooking surfaces for allergen-free foods. Label containers clearly, and implement strict cleaning routines to avoid any accidental exposure. Be especially cautious when preparing meals for both allergic and non-allergic individuals in the same household.

Allergen-Free Recipes: Explore allergen-free recipes that align with your anti-inflammatory goals. Many cookbooks and online resources focus on allergen-free, anti-inflammatory diets, providing a wealth of creative ideas to keep your meals interesting and nutritious.

Stay Informed: Stay updated on the latest information about food allergies, allergen labeling laws, and emerging allergens. Awareness of regulatory changes and new research can help you make informed decisions. Regularly review food safety guidelines to stay proactive in managing your condition.

Carry an Epinephrine Auto-Injector: If you have severe food allergies that can lead to anaphylaxis, always carry an epinephrine auto-injector. Ensure that you, your family, friends, and coworkers know how to use it in case of an emergency. Regularly check the expiration date of your auto-injector and replace it as needed.

Allergen-Free Dining Apps: Consider using allergen-free dining apps or websites that help identify restaurants and dishes catering to specific allergens. These tools often provide user reviews, allergen menus, and recommendations, making it easier to find safe dining options, especially when traveling.

Support Groups: Join food allergy support groups or online communities. Connecting with others who share similar experiences can provide emotional support, practical advice, and tips for managing daily challenges. Support groups can also be valuable resources for discovering new allergen-free products and recipes.

Seek Medical Advice: Consult with a healthcare professional or allergist to confirm your allergies, receive personalized guidance, and discuss any dietary restrictions. Regular check-ups and allergy tests can help monitor your condition and adjust your management plan as needed.

Dealing with food allergies while following an anti-inflammatory diet requires extra diligence, but it is entirely manageable. Being well-informed, communicating your needs, and paying attention to labels and ingredients can help you maintain a healthy, anti-inflammatory lifestyle while safeguarding against allergens.

Budget-Friendly Anti-Inflammatory Eating

Eating an anti-inflammatory diet doesn't have to break the bank. With a bit of planning and savvy shopping, you can make choices that are both healthy and budget-friendly. Here are some tips for incorporating anti-inflammatory foods without straining your wallet:

Buy in Bulk: Purchasing non-perishable anti-inflammatory staples in bulk can save you money in the long run. This includes items like rice, quinoa, dried beans, oats, and spices. Buying in larger quantities often reduces the cost per unit, making it an economical option. Store these items properly in airtight containers to maintain freshness.

Seasonal and Local Produce: Seasonal and locally grown fruits and vegetables are often more affordable and fresher than their out-of-season counterparts. Visit farmers' markets, local farms, or join a community-supported agriculture (CSA) program to access cost-effective, fresh produce. Seasonal produce also tends to be at its peak flavor and nutritional value.

Frozen Fruits and Vegetables: Frozen fruits and vegetables are a budget-friendly alternative to fresh produce. They are usually flash-frozen at their peak ripeness, retaining their nutritional value. Frozen options are convenient for smoothies, stir-fries, soups, and stews. They also have a longer shelf life, reducing the risk of food waste.

Canned or Dried Legumes: Canned or dried legumes, such as chickpeas, lentils, and black beans, are cost-effective sources of plant-based protein. They're versatile and can be used in soups, salads, stews, and dips like hummus. Dried legumes are even more economical than canned ones, though they require soaking and longer cooking times.

Affordable Protein Sources: Opt for budget-friendly protein sources like eggs, canned tuna, and lean cuts of meat or poultry when they're on sale. Incorporate these proteins into balanced meals with vegetables and whole grains.

Buying larger portions of meat and freezing them in smaller servings can also save money.

Make Homemade: Cooking at home allows you to control ingredients and costs. Make your own soups, sauces, salad dressings, and snacks instead of buying pre-made versions. Batch cooking and meal prepping can help you save both time and money while ensuring healthier meal options.

Embrace Whole Grains: Choose whole grains like brown rice, oats, and whole wheat pasta. They're more affordable than many specialty health foods and provide more nutrients than refined grains. Buying in bulk can further reduce costs, and these grains have a long shelf life when stored properly.

Limit Processed Foods: Processed foods are often more expensive and less nutritious. Minimize your consumption of packaged snacks, ready-to-eat meals, and sugary beverages. Instead, focus on whole, minimally processed foods that offer better value for your health and budget.

Reduce Meat Consumption: Consider adopting meatless meals a few times a week. Plant-based proteins like beans, lentils, tofu, and tempeh are economical, nutrient-dense, and environmentally friendly. Incorporate dishes like vegetable stir-fries, lentil soups, and bean salads into your meal rotation.

Plan Meals and Use Leftovers: Plan your meals for the week and create a shopping list to avoid impulse purchases. Cooking in batches and using leftovers creatively can reduce food waste and save money. Repurpose leftovers into new dishes, such as turning roasted vegetables into a hearty soup.

Opt for Generic Brands: Generic or store-brand products are usually less expensive than name brands but still offer comparable quality. Compare ingredient lists to ensure you're getting the same nutritional value at a lower cost.

Purchase Non-Perishables Online: Look for deals on non-perishable anti-inflammatory items online. Many online retailers offer competitive prices, bulk discounts, and subscription services that can be cost-effective. Compare prices across platforms to find the best deals.

Store Food Properly: Properly storing your food can prevent spoilage and extend its shelf life. Use airtight containers, refrigerate or freeze perishable items promptly, and practice "first in, first out" rotation to use older items before newer ones.

Coupon and Sale Alerts: Sign up for coupon websites, grocery store loyalty programs, or use apps that notify you of sales, discounts, and special offers at your local grocery stores. Taking advantage of these deals can significantly reduce your grocery bill over time.

Buy Whole Foods: Whole foods like fruits, vegetables, and grains are often more affordable than pre-cut, pre-packaged, or convenience versions. Preparing these foods yourself not only saves money but also ensures you're consuming fresher, less processed options.

By implementing these budget-friendly strategies, you can enjoy the benefits of an anti-inflammatory diet without overspending. Thoughtful planning, smart shopping, and home cooking are key to maintaining both your health and your budget.

Sustainability and Eco-Friendly Choices

Eating in an anti-inflammatory way not only benefits your health but can also have a positive impact on the environment. Sustainable and eco-friendly choices can reduce your carbon footprint and contribute to a healthier planet. Here are some ways to align your anti-inflammatory diet with eco-conscious decisions:

Choose Local and Seasonal Produce: Opt for fruits and vegetables that are in season and locally grown. This reduces the energy and resources required for transportation and storage, supports local farmers, and often results in fresher, more nutrient-dense produce.

Reduce Meat Consumption: Reducing your meat consumption or opting for plant-based proteins like beans, lentils, and legumes can significantly lower your environmental impact. The meat industry has a substantial carbon footprint due to greenhouse gas emissions, land use, and water consumption.

Buy Organic When Possible: Organic foods are grown with fewer synthetic pesticides and chemicals, which benefits both your health and the environment. Organic farming practices often promote soil health, biodiversity, and reduce pollution from agricultural runoff.

Minimize Food Waste: Plan your meals, store food properly, and use leftovers creatively to minimize food waste. Composting food scraps can further reduce your environmental impact by diverting waste from landfills and enriching the soil.

Support Sustainable Seafood: When choosing seafood, look for options that are sustainably sourced, such as those certified by the Marine Stewardship Council (MSC). Sustainable fishing practices help protect marine ecosystems and maintain fish populations.

Choose Eco-Friendly Packaging: Opt for products with minimal, recyclable, or biodegradable packaging to reduce plastic waste. Buying in bulk can also help decrease the amount of packaging used, leading to less waste overall.

Use Reusable Bags and Containers: Reduce your reliance on single-use plastics by using reusable shopping bags, water bottles, and food containers. This simple habit can significantly cut down on plastic pollution.

Reduce Food Miles: Select foods with lower "food miles," meaning they have traveled a shorter distance from farm to plate. This reduces energy consumption and emissions associated with long-distance transportation.

Grow Your Own: If you have the space and resources, consider starting a home garden. Growing your own herbs, fruits, and vegetables can be both satisfying and sustainable, reducing your reliance on store-bought produce.

Be Mindful of Water Usage: Conserve water when cooking and cleaning, and consider the environmental impact of water-intensive foods, such as almonds and avocados. Simple practices like using a dishwasher efficiently or reusing cooking water can help save water.

Choose Sustainable Cooking Methods: When preparing meals, consider energy-efficient cooking methods like steaming, stir-frying, or using a pressure cooker. These methods use less energy and often preserve more nutrients in your food.

Support Sustainable Brands: Choose food brands and companies that prioritize sustainability, ethical sourcing, and eco-friendly practices. Supporting such brands encourages more businesses to adopt environmentally responsible practices.

Reduce Single-Use Plastics: Cut back on single-use plastics like disposable utensils, straws, and water bottles. Opt for durable, reusable alternatives made from stainless steel, glass, or bamboo.

Educate Yourself: Stay informed about the environmental impact of different foods and dietary choices. Knowledge empowers you to make more eco-friendly decisions and advocate for sustainable food systems.

Reduce Energy Consumption: Lower your energy consumption by using energy-efficient appliances, cooking with lids on pots to retain heat, and turning off kitchen devices when not in use.

Join Eco-Friendly Movements: Consider joining or supporting initiatives and movements that promote sustainable and eco-friendly eating practices. Community-supported agriculture (CSA), zero-waste groups, and local environmental organizations can provide resources and inspiration.

By incorporating sustainable and eco-friendly choices into your anti-inflammatory diet, you not only benefit your health but also contribute to the well-being of the planet. Small changes in your food choices and habits can collectively make a significant impact on the environment.

Chapter 7: Resources and References

Websites and Apps

Here are some trusted websites and apps that provide valuable information, practical tools, and guidance to help you maintain an anti-inflammatory diet effectively.

Websites	URL
PubMed A comprehensive database of scientific articles and clinical studies covering a wide range of health topics, including inflammation, nutrition, and chronic diseases. It's an excellent resource for accessing peer-reviewed research and the latest scientific findings on anti-inflammatory diets.	
National Center for Complementary and Integrative Health A U.S. government agency that provides evidence-based information on complementary and integrative health approaches, including dietary supplements, herbal remedies, and nutrition. It offers research updates and guidance on how these approaches impact inflammation and overall health.	
Arthritis Foundation A leading organization dedicated to supporting individuals with arthritis and related inflammatory conditions. The site offers practical tips, meal plans, and evidence-based recommendations for reducing inflammation through diet, exercise, and lifestyle changes.	
Harvard Health Publishing A trusted source of health information from Harvard Medical School. The site features articles, guides, and expert insights on nutrition science, the role of inflammation in chronic diseases, and evidence-based dietary recommendations to promote long-term health.	
Centers for Disease Control and Prevention The CDC offers comprehensive guidelines on nutrition, physical activity, and chronic disease prevention. Its resources include dietary recommendations, tips for healthy living, and evidence-based strategies to reduce inflammation and support overall well-being.	
National Health Service The NHS provides clear, practical advice on healthy eating, nutrition, and managing chronic health conditions. Its resources are grounded in scientific evidence and include dietary guidelines that support an anti-inflammatory lifestyle.	

Apps for Smartphones	App Store	Google Play
MyFitnessPal • Track everything you eat to monitor your daily food intake. • Monitor your calorie consumption to help manage your diet. • Analyze the balance of proteins, fats, and carbohydrates in your meals. • Keep a record of your daily water intake to ensure proper hydration. • Log your physical activities and workouts to track calories burned.		
OurGroceries • Share and sync grocery lists in real-time across multiple devices. • Add photos or notes to items for accurate product selection. • Use voice assistants like Alexa, Siri, or Google Assistant to add items. • Save recipes and add all ingredients to shopping lists with one tap. • Organize shopping lists automatically by categories or aisles.		
Mealime • Create personalized meal plans based on dietary preferences and restrictions. • Generate organized grocery lists from selected recipes for easy shopping. • Send grocery lists to fulfillment partners for quick online ordering. • Follow step-by-step cooking instructions to prepare meals in 30 minutes or less. • Reduce food waste with meal plans designed to use ingredients efficiently.		
Gut Health • Provides anti-inflammatory recipes designed to support gut health. • Offers personalized diet plans to maintain a balanced gut microbiome. • Tracks gut health progress and helps manage digestive issues effectively. • Includes a comprehensive list of antioxidant-rich foods and probiotics. • Allows saving favorite recipes and accessing articles on gut health and nutrition.		

Further Assistance

If you have additional questions or need further guidance on your anti-inflammatory journey, don't hesitate to seek help from the following sources:

Registered Dietitians and Nutritionists: These professionals are experts in dietary guidance and can provide personalized recommendations tailored to your specific needs and goals. They can help you create meal plans, address dietary restrictions, and monitor your progress.

Healthcare Providers: Consult with your healthcare provider for personalized advice, especially if you have specific medical conditions or dietary requirements. They can offer guidance that takes your overall health into account.

Support Groups: Joining or seeking support from anti-inflammatory or healthy eating support groups can provide valuable insights, motivation, and a sense of community. You can often find such groups locally or online.

Health and Wellness Coaches: These professionals specialize in guiding individuals toward healthier lifestyles. They can help you set and achieve your dietary and wellness goals.

Local Farmers' Markets: Farmers' markets can be great places to connect with local growers and food producers. They often provide information on seasonal, fresh, and locally sourced products that can align with an anti-inflammatory diet.

Holistic Health Practitioners: Holistic health practitioners may incorporate dietary guidance and alternative therapies to promote overall well-being. Consult with one if you're interested in a holistic approach to health.

Allergists: If you have food allergies, allergists can help you identify and manage your allergies while adhering to an anti-inflammatory diet.

Online Communities: Explore online forums and communities focused on anti-inflammatory living, nutrition, and wellness. These communities can provide additional insights and support from individuals with similar goals.

Cookbooks: Explore a wide range of anti-inflammatory cookbooks to find inspiration, recipes, and meal planning ideas. Cookbooks often offer practical advice and insights into preparing anti-inflammatory dishes.

Nutritional Analysis Tools: Use nutritional analysis tools and software to track your dietary intake and assess your nutrient consumption. Some apps and websites offer these features to help you monitor your diet more effectively.

Educational Courses: Consider enrolling in online or in-person educational courses related to nutrition, cooking, or anti-inflammatory living. These courses can provide structured learning and hands-on experience.

Remember that seeking assistance is a sign of proactive self-care. These resources and professionals are available to support you on your anti-inflammatory journey, helping you navigate the dietary changes and lifestyle adjustments with confidence.

Conclusion

As you reach the end of this book, it's essential to acknowledge and celebrate the progress you've made on your anti-inflammatory journey. Whether you've just started or have been following this lifestyle for a while, each step you've taken is a significant accomplishment. Here are a few ways to celebrate your journey and stay motivated:

Reflect on Your Achievements: Take a moment to reflect on how far you've come. Consider the positive changes you've made in your diet, lifestyle, and health.

Share Your Success: Share your journey with friends and family. Your experience can inspire others to make healthier choices too.

Set New Goals: Consider setting new goals to continue your anti-inflammatory lifestyle. These goals can be related to dietary improvements, exercise, or other aspects of wellness.

Treat Yourself: Celebrate with a treat that aligns with your anti-inflammatory diet. Enjoy a special meal or a delicious homemade anti-inflammatory dessert.

Practice Gratitude: Cultivate a sense of gratitude for your body's ability to heal and adapt. Recognize the importance of self-care.

Keep Learning: Continue to expand your knowledge about nutrition, health, and wellness. Stay curious and open to new information and discoveries.

Stay Connected: Stay connected with the resources and communities that have supported you on your journey. These connections can provide ongoing encouragement and assistance.

Be Kind to Yourself: Remember that setbacks and challenges are a normal part of any journey. Be kind to yourself and view these moments as opportunities to learn and grow.

Embrace Balance: Balance is key to long-term success. Enjoy your anti-inflammatory lifestyle without becoming overly rigid. Flexibility allows for both health and happiness.

Celebrate Small Wins: Celebrate not only major milestones but also the small victories along the way. Each choice you make contributes to your well-being.

Your anti-inflammatory journey is a lifelong commitment to health and well-being. By taking the initiative to make positive changes, you're investing in a future full of vitality, balance, and joy. So, celebrate your journey, be proud of your efforts, and continue to explore the boundless potential of an anti-inflammatory lifestyle. Your health and happiness are worth every step you take.

Appendices

Glossary of Anti-Inflammatory Terms

Here are some key terms and phrases frequently used in the context of an anti-inflammatory diet:

Inflammation: The body's natural response to injury, infection, or harm. It can be acute or chronic and plays a role in many diseases.

Anti-Inflammatory: Refers to foods, practices, or substances that help reduce inflammation in the body.

Cytokines: Proteins produced by cells in the body, including the immune system, that regulate inflammation and immune responses.

Omega-3 Fatty Acids: A type of polyunsaturated fat found in certain foods, particularly in fatty fish like salmon and flaxseeds, known for their anti-inflammatory properties.

Antioxidants: Compounds that help protect the body from oxidative stress and reduce inflammation. They are abundant in fruits, vegetables, and certain spices.

Polyphenols: Naturally occurring compounds found in plant foods, such as green tea and berries, known for their anti-inflammatory and antioxidant effects.

Probiotics: Live beneficial bacteria that support gut health and the immune system, potentially reducing inflammation.

Prebiotics: Non-digestible fibers that nourish the beneficial bacteria in the gut, promoting a healthy microbiome.

Glycemic Index (GI): A ranking of how quickly a carbohydrate-containing food raises blood sugar levels.Foods with a lower GI are less likely to cause inflammation.

Whole Foods: Foods that are minimally processed and close to their natural state. These include fruits, vegetables, whole grains, and unprocessed meats.

Plant-Based Diet: A diet primarily composed of plant-based foods, such as fruits, vegetables, nuts, seeds, and grains, known for their anti-inflammatory properties.

Gluten: A protein found in wheat, barley, rye, and their derivatives. Some individuals have gluten sensitivities that can lead to inflammation.

Leaky Gut Syndrome: A condition in which the lining of the intestine becomes damaged, potentially allowing toxins and bacteria to enter the bloodstream, leading to inflammation.

Elimination Diet: A dietary approach that involves removing certain foods or food groups, such as potential allergens or inflammatory triggers, to identify specific dietary sensitivities.

Food Allergy: An adverse immune response to specific foods, which can lead to inflammation and various symptoms.

Mindful Eating: A practice of paying full attention to the experience of eating, which can lead to healthier choices and better digestion.

Curcumin: The active compound in turmeric, known for its anti-inflammatory and antioxidant effects.

Adaptogens: Herbs or substances that may help the body adapt to stress and reduce inflammation

Measurement Conversion Charts

Conversion charts can be invaluable when working with recipes or dietary guidelines that use different measurement systems. Here are some common measurement conversions to help you navigate your anti-inflammatory diet with ease:

Volume Conversions:

- **1 tablespoon (tbsp)** = 3 teaspoons (tsp)
- **1 fluid ounce (fl oz)** = 2 tablespoons
- **1 cup** = 8 fluid ounces
- **1 pint (pt)** = 2 cups, **1 quart (qt)** = 4 cups

Weight Conversions:

- **1 ounce (oz)** = 28.35 grams (g)
- **1 pound (lb)** = 16 ounces
- **1 kilogram (kg)** = 2.205 pounds

Metric to Imperial Conversions:

- **1 milliliter (ml)** = 0.034 fluid ounces
- **1 liter (L)** = 1.76 pints
- **1 gram (g)** = 0.035 ounces
- **1 kilogram (kg)** = 2.2 pounds

Temperature Conversions:

- Fahrenheit (°F) to Celsius (°C): (°F - 32) × 5/9 (e.g., 350°F = 180°C)
- Celsius (°C) to Fahrenheit (°F): (°C × 9/5) + 32

Oven Temperature Conversions:

- Very slow oven: **250°F or 120°C**
- Slow oven: **300°F or 150°C**
- Moderate oven: **350°F or 180°C**
- Moderately hot oven: **375°F or 190°C**
- Hot oven: **400°F or 200°C**
- Very hot oven: **450°F or 230°C**

Common Kitchen Conversions:

- **1 teaspoon (tsp)** = 5 milliliters (ml)
- **1 tablespoon (tbsp)** = 15 milliliters (ml)
- **1 cup** = 240 milliliters (ml)
- **1/4 cup** = 60 ml, **1/2 cup** = 120 ml, **3/4 cup** = 180 ml

These conversion charts can be handy references when you come across recipes or dietary guidelines using different measurements. Whether you're following a recipe from a different region or converting nutrition labels, these charts will help ensure accurate and consistent measurements.

Personal Notes

Made in United States
Orlando, FL
03 May 2025

60966868R10063